HEALTH SECTOR REFORMS IN INDIA

Centre de Sciences Humaines (Centre for Social Sciences and Humanities): Created in 1989 and based in New Delhi, the CSH is part of the network of research centres of the French Ministry of Foreign Affairs. The Centre's research work is primarily oriented towards the study of issues concerning the contemporary dynamics of development in India and South Asia. The activities of the Centre are focused on four main themes, namely: Economic growth and sustainable development, International and regional relations, Institutional structures and political constructions of identity and Urban dynamics.

Centre de Sciences Humaines, 2, Aurangzeb Road, New Delhi 110011, India, Tel: (91) 11 3041 00 70, Fax: (91 11) 3041 00 79
E-mail: infos@csh-delhi.com
Website: http://www.csh-delhi.com

Institut Français de Pondichéry (French Institute of Pondicherry): Created in 1955, the IFP is a multidisciplinary research and advanced educational institute. Major research works are focusing on Sanskrit and Tamil languages and literatures—in close collaboration with the Ecole Française d'Extrême-Orient—ecosystems, biodiversity and sustainability, dynamics of population and socio-economic development.

Institut Français de Pondichéry, 11, Saint Louis Street, PB 33
Pondicherry 605001, Tel: (91) 413 2334 168
Fax: (91) 413 2339 534
E-mail: ifpdir@ifpindia.org

HEALTH SECTOR REFORMS IN INDIA

Edited by

GIRISH KUMAR

MANOHAR

CENTRE DE SCIENCES HUMAINES

2009

First published 2009

ISBN 978-81-7304-811-1

Published by

Ajay Kumar Jain *for*
Manohar Publishers & Distributors
4753/23 Ansari Road, Daryaganj
New Delhi 110 002

Typeset at

Digigrafics
New Delhi 110 049

Printed at

Salasar Imaging Systems
Delhi 110 035

Contents

Preface

All this started with a half-page story on the renovation of an Indore-based associate hospital of a medical college of British vintage, then in the throes of an unprecedented crisis. The highlight of the story (*India Today*, 8 January 2001: 9) was the innovative way in which the crisis was handled by the then district collector. In this gigantic task, he relied on people's contribution alone (without taking recourse to the district treasury) and a working model of participatory management structure for its upkeep once the hospital was refurbished and given a new lease of life. This short report was impressive by all accounts. It triggered a chain of thought in my mind (what I had earlier read about or heard of from both serving and retired civil servants) recalling innovative projects worked out by district collectors in so many towns/cities across the states over the past years. Sustainability aspects of such projects were quite often questioned because of neglect. For, once their progenitors were transferred, their successors simply wouldn't have the time or the inclination to follow up on his/her predecessor's brainchild. This was the reason that held me back, though I was keen to personally witness the changes brought out into the functioning of the MY Hospital. Aware that the model was to be replicated in every district and tahsil-level hospital across the state of Madhya Pradesh, I approached all those I knew in the state to identify just one hospital where the lead was taken by an insider, a doctor serving that hospital itself. I singled out one hospital since I was then involved in a major project on another subject, therefore I was not sure whether I would have the time and resources to study so many hospitals, if named by my acquaintances.

Six months later, I was told about the Badnagar Tahsil Hospital where the progenitor was none other than its chief medical officer, Dr. L.A. Kapadia, a noted general surgeon of the region.

Month upon month rolled by but I could not find the time to do anything on this project except locate the tahsil on the state map and make a few phone calls to the concerned doctor.

It was on a winter afternoon (January 2002) that I finally reached Badnagar, a nondescript small town, located at a distance of nearly 50 km from Ujjain, the headquarters of the district bearing the same name, otherwise known as an ancient temple town. During the next twenty-four hours of my stay there, I must have met more than 100-odd people, in and around Badnagar Hospital. This included doctors, paramedics, patients, their attendants and curious onlookers as well as local journalists, government officials and elected representatives. On my way back, following this exhaustive but most satisfying short visit, I was again in a quandary: should I write about the unique experiences of Badnagar Hospital? The persisting dilemma was that it could have been a case of most unusual, exceptional reform triggered by local circumstances. At the most, the credit goes to a doctor who, with the help of some good Samaritans, changed adversity into a great opportunity. But would it last once the doctor who was at the centre of the entire reform process and structure was gone? A meeting with the then Chief Medical Officer of Ujjain District Hospital (administrative controller of Badnagar Hospital) on my way back to Bhopal cleared my all lingering doubts.

Finally, I wrote about the success story of Badnagar Hospital (*Economic & Political Weekly*, 19 July 2003, pp. 3041-5). One disconcerting question, however, remained on my mind: had the initiatives taken by the then collector of Indore heralded institutional reforms in Madhya Pradesh hospitals? This was not possible to answer without micro level study of a fairly large number of hospitals at different levels, selected from different districts. It required a modest budget and also a suitable time frame. Both my worries were sorted out by the Delhi-based French research institute, the Centre de Sciences Humaines (CSH), of which I had already become a part since early 2001.

I am, therefore, beholden to Dr. Frederic Grare, the then Director of CSH. Not only did he encourage me to undertake this study and provide the financial resources required for the purpose but, in view of my engagements in other projects, Dr. Grare also allowed me to have a staggered time schedule for the project, to be taken up as a case study. I am also grateful to his successor, Dr. Veronique Dupont, who prompted me to expand my engagements with the health sector by organizing a national seminar on the subject. This was eventually organized, thanks to the additional financial support extended by the Indian Council of Social Science Research (New Delhi), within the broad rubric of an Indo-French bilateral agreement on social science research.

From identifying contributors on state-specific health reforms to certain other vital aspects of seminar coordination, the person who helped me immensely was Dr. Rama V. Baru, an old hand on the subject from the Centre for Social Medicine and Community Health (CSMCH), JNU (New Delhi) to whom I am most grateful. I am thankful to several of her colleagues from the centre for participating in the seminar and enhancing the quality of debate through their informed interventions. My sincere thanks are also due to several senior colleagues, well-wishers who happily honoured my request to either chair sessions or act as discussants. Included in this list are Professor Manoranjan Mohanty presently a Professor at Council for Social Development, New Delhi), Professor Amitabh Kundu (Dean, School of Social Sciences, JNU), Professor Ritu Priya (CSMCH/JNU), Professor Amit Shovan Ray (School of International Studies/JNU), Professor Ghanshyam Shah (formerly of CSMCH), Professor Moneer Alam (Institute of Economic Growth, Delhi), Dr. A.B. Dey (Professor of Medicine, All India Institute of Medical Sciences, New Delhi), Dr. K.C. George (Director, Institute of Health Management, Hyderabad), and Dr. George Mathew (Director, Institute of Social Sciences, New Delhi).

For delivering the keynote addresses, I am grateful to Professor Balbir Arora (then Rector, JNU) and Ms. Sushma Chowdhury, (then Advisor, Health, Family Welfare & Nutrition, Planning Commission), a retired IAS officer of Jammu & Kashmir cadre—meeting her was akin to a rediscovery after a gap of more than fifteen years since I had met her last in Kashmir. Above all, I am indebted to Dr. Binayak Sen, a medical doctor working among the tribals, combining his role as health-cum-human rights activist, who came all the way from Raipur to discuss what was happening in Chhattisgarh.

I also owe a word of special appreciation to Mr. N.R. Mohanty, former collector of Indore whose intervention heralded public hospital reforms in Madhya Pradesh, who patiently shared his experiences and helped me otherwise. My thanks are also due to Mr. Pravir Krishn, another IAS officer of Madhya Pradesh cadre, presently Joint Secretary, Ministry of Health and Family Welfare, who was a real support in the course of my work in Madhya Pradesh and also for clearing my doubts on the administrative aspects of public institutions. I also thankfully acknowledge the cooperation received from Dr. Arun P. Bali, Director (International Cooperation), ICSSR, towards conducting the seminar.

My special thanks are also due to all those who presented or sent their papers for the seminar. All the more for waiting patiently to find their paper included in the volume which, for a variety of reasons, has taken much more time than I had initially anticipated. I wish to gratefully acknowledge the general editorial guidance received from Manohar Publishers, particularly of Mr. Siddharth Chowdhury, for making the volume more reader-friendly. Finally, I thankfully acknowledge the continued institutional interest of the CSH as displayed by its present Director, Dr. Basudeb Chaudhuri, and its Publications-in-charge, Ms. Rupa Sengupta and her successor Ms. Arpita Mitra, towards this endeavour. I am equally grateful to Mr. B.S. Baswan, Director of IIPA, for his affable support in taking this unfinished task to its logical conclusion.

In the end, I wish to put on record my special gratitude to my wife, Rumjhum, a.k.a. Mrs. Rakshita Verma, who ungrudgingly allowed me the long working hours required to give shape to this work.

New Delhi GIRISH KUMAR
24 March 2009

Contributors

RAMA V. BARU is Associate Professor at Centre for Social Medicine and Community Health, JNU, New Delhi.

LALITA DESAI is Founder Member and Managing Trustee of SEWA Rural Trust.

JOY ELAMON is a medical doctor cum public health activist working with Swiss Agency for Development and Cooperation (SDC) as the Chief Programme Coordinator, CapDecK (Programme on Capacity Development for Decentralisation in Kerala).

BUDDHADEB GHOSH is a Senior Fellow at the Institute of Social Sciences, New Delhi. Earlier, he served the Government of West Bengal in various capacities, including a stint as Director, State Institute of Panchayats, Kalyani.

GIRISH KUMAR is Senior Fellow at Indian Institute of Public Administration, New Delhi. Earlier, he was Senior Fellow and Head, Political Science Division of Centre de Sciences Humaines, New Delhi.

SUBRATA KUNDU is currently a Visiting Fellow at Centre for Public Policy, Indian Institute of Management, Bangalore. He completed his Ph.D. in Public Health from Jawaharlal Nehru University, New Delhi in 2006.

N. LALITHA is Associate Professor, Gujarat Institute of Development Research, Ahmedabad.

SUBRATA K. MONDAL is an economist who earlier worked on projects undertaken by NCAER. He is presently associated with a Ranchi-based NGO.

BINAYAK SEN is a medical doctor working for long as health-cum-human rights activist among the tribals in Chhattisgarh.

PANKAJ SHAH is Director, Community Health Programme, SEWA-Rural, Jhagadia (Bharuch), Gujarat.

SHOBHA SHAH is Coordinator, Resource & Training Centre, SEWA-Rural, Jhagadia (Bharuch), Gujarat.

ABUSALEH SHARIFF is Senior Research Fellow at the New Delhi office of International Food Policy Research Institute (IFPRI). Prior to joining IFPRI he was Chief Economist at the National Council of Applied Economics Research, New Delhi.

ALAIN VAGUET is Associate Professor of Geography, University of Rouen, France.

CHAPTER 1

Introduction Health Sector Reforms in India: Issues, Experiences and Trends

GIRISH KUMAR

BACKGROUND

The last decade of the twentieth century heralded a new beginning in the country. First and foremost was the unfolding of economic policy reforms initiated in early 1991. Although the reforms were targeted mainly at the core sectors of commerce, finance and industry, the policy measures triggered a chain of actions leading to deregulation and privatization in other areas. This *inter alia* assured a recognized space for the private sector to operate in the areas till then considered to be exclusive preserves of the public sector. Second, the 73rd and 74th Constitutional Amendments (1992) brought a comprehensive decentralization package, also paving way for community initiatives at the local level. Although the political regimes both in the Centre and the provinces/states have been criticized for the sluggish pace of reforms, the post-liberalization phase has offered ample scope for restructuring the pattern of governance. This entails creating democratic space and laying enabling conditions by the state for participation of the people in managing their affairs at the local level. Steps taken in that direction, it was assumed, would facilitate both private as well as community initiatives in the public domain, largely monopolized by ineffective state institutions.

In the health sector, the implications of ineffective state institutions meant: absence or near-absence of medico and para-medico personnel in remote areas, negligence on the part of health bureaucracy and medico personnel alike, and lack of infrastructure including unavailability of Primary Health Centres (PHC) and Sub-Health Centres (SHC) in required numbers in the rural areas. This is not to deny that a massive expansion of rural health infrastructure[1] had already been undertaken during the period of Sixth (1982-7) and Seventh Five Year (1987-92) Plans. But studies conducted during the second half of the Seventh Plan and also during the initial years of the Eighth Plan period had revealed that PHCs were 'grossly underutilized' largely due to inadequate 'staff, medicine, equipment, transport, etc.', and also because the PHCs were mainly engaged in 'completing family planning[2] targets' (Duggal, Nandraj and Vadir, 1995).

Under the given circumstances the rural populace was left with no other option except turn to private practitioners, quite often trained in non-allopathic systems, or flock to already crowded taluka/block (sub-district) or district level hospitals. What aggravated the matter further was the progressive reduction in budgetary allocations in the health sector.[3] This was in conformity with the World Bank's agenda for the health sector. It needs mentioning that with the Eighth Five Year Plan, the Union Government had already agreed to accept the major recommendations of the World Bank. This included budgetary cuts in public spending on health services, introduction of 'user fee' and privatization of medical care (Qadeer, 1999; Rao, 1999; Krishnan, 1999; World Bank, 1993). To cap it all, it is estimated that nearly three-fourths (about 70 per cent) of the total health budget in most of the states is spent on meeting recurring expenditure on salaries and establishment alone. In plain words, the reduction in health allocations has greatly affected the non-salary components of the health expenditure.

SHRINKING INVESTMENT

There was substantial investment in the social sector in the 1950s and 1960s, the first two decades after India's independence. The tempo could not be maintained in the 1970s in the wake of the oil crisis, which triggered a worldwide recession. In fact, 'the late 1970s saw a cut-back of investments in the social sectors and the debate on privatization gained importance' in the developed world primarily, though it had wider ramifications for the developing countries, including India (Baru, 1998; Nandraj, Muraleedharan et al., 2001). Following the initiation of economic reforms in 1991, it was envisaged that the gradual withdrawal of the federal government from the public sector (read industry mainly and to some extent infrastructure, too) would enable it to hike its spending in the social sector. Contrary to this perceived wisdom, the fiscal situation deteriorated, 'following a temporary stabilization in the early 1990s, eroding the government's ability to step up investments in health'. Notwithstanding this fact, allocation for Centrally sponsored health programmes continued to increase, up from Rs. 208.17 crore in 1992-3 to Rs. 489.71 crore in 1996-7, thanks to external assistance from both bilateral and multilateral sources (Misra, et al., 2003: 30). Another point to be considered, which is rather more significant, is that the share of the state governments accounts for 75 per cent of total public health expenditure. What matters more, therefore, is the financial health of states than that of the Centre. And most of the state governments suffer from acute fiscal deficits. The stated reasons are many, including the states' inability to cut subsidies, privatize loss-making public undertakings, curtail the oversized bureaucracy etc.[4] It requires mentioning here that the fiscal crisis faced by the states was further aggravated by a sharp increase in the salary and pension bills in the wake of the Fifth Pay Commission's recommendations. All these have resulted in 'sharp reductions in the non-salary recurring expenditure in public health facilities' (ibid.).

In any case, the public health expenditure in India is one of the lowest in the world, less than 1 per cent (0.90 per cent to be precise) of its GDP. As a matter of fact, of the total health expenditure in India, only 15 per cent is public expenditure,[5] the rest is private expenditure.[6] Apparently, the investment in health sector has gone down over the years, adversely affecting health care of the poor and marginalized sections of the society. To understand its implications some illustrations are required.

Health status of children: According to the 1998-9 National Family Health Survey, 'Half of all Indian children are undernourished[7] and half of all adult women suffer anaemia. At the time of the survey, 30 per cent of all children under the age of three had fever, another 20 per cent had diarrhoea, and another 20 per cent had symptoms of acute respiratory infection. . . . Half of all Indian children below three suffer from one of these conditions at any given point of time.' This is, however, not to overlook the success of health care in India. For instance, polio eradication campaign and due to certain other immunization programmes, smallpox has almost been eradicated. To some extent this is true of leprosy too. Thanks to vaccinations of different types, the frequent outbreak of communicable diseases has become a matter of past.

Scanty infrastructure: A little over two-thirds (69 per cent) of PHCs have one bed, one-fifth is equipped with telephone facility and 12 per cent indulge in the luxury of regular maintenance. These aggregate figures are national averages which do not tell us the worst type of variations at the state level and below. A great majority of PHCs in Bihar, for instance, make do 'without electricity, a weighing machine or even a toilet' (Dreze, 2004).

State-wise variations: The significance of good public health facilities has been recognized by only a few states such as Himachal Pradesh, Kerala, and Tamil Nadu. Having visited a large number of PHCs in three districts of Tamil Nadu, Dreze (2004) observed:

> The PHCs in Tamil Nadu were clean, lively and well staffed. Plenty of medicines were available for free, and there were regular inspections. The walls were plastered with charts and posters giving details of daily routine, available facilities, progress of various programmes, and related information. Patients streamed in and out, evidently at ease with the system. It was a joy to see this, in contrast with the bare, deserted, gloomy, hostile premises that pass for health centres in north India.

No wonder, in Tamil Nadu, practically all births are preceded by antenatal check-ups and 89 per cent children are fully vaccinated (Dreze, 2004). The corresponding figures in UP are 35 and 21 per cent. The health indicators of bigger states like UP and MP are 'at the level of Sub-Saharan Africa' (Jalan, 2004).

Utilisation pattern: 'Absence of health workers range between 35 and 58 per cent in different Indian states. At a district-level study in Udaipur (Rajasthan), for instance, 'more than half of the health sub-centres were found to be closed during regular opening hours.' It was a little over one-third (36 per cent precisely) at the level of PHCs and CHCs (Dreze, 2004).

Multiple agencies and overlapping functions: With multiple functions to discharge, the Union Ministry of Health has virtually no control over its line departments/organizations. 'There is an overlap of functions with conflicting objectives among different ministries involved in health care. The Ministry of Chemicals and Fertilizer, for instance, 'is responsible for the regulation, licensing, and price control of drugs. The Ministry of Health, on the other hand, is responsible for ensuring the availability of good-quality drugs in all parts of the country'. The former, as part of its policy to promote industry, allocated license to 20,000 small units to manufacture drugs, 'but it has had highly adverse consequences for the quality of drugs, because smaller units have been unable to provide the infrastructure for quality control' (Jalan, 2004).

Ruthless profiteers: While the public health care is highly insufficient, the 'private services[8] are virtually unregulated, leaving patients at the mercy of unscrupulous practitioners. Fraud, overmedication and unnecessary surgery'[9] happen to be the hallmark of private health care. In fact, the spurt in private health care has led to further dichotomy in the society. A major chunk of the population cannot afford the cost of the services available in the private sector. Consequently, 'the number of people who could not seek medical care because of lack of money has increased between 1986 and 1995. The proportion of people unable to afford[10] basic health care has doubled in last decade. . . . Over 20 million Indians are pushed below poverty line every year because of the effect of out of pocket spending on health care' (Deogaonkar, 2005).

FROM 1950s TO 1980s: U-TURN IN HEALTH CARE

In post-Independence India what initially started as a programme for eradicating malaria and small pox, resulted in a huge infrastructure of public health in the 1950s and 1960s. During the

1960s and 1970s primary-level health services grew, largely due to the pumping of funds for the 'vertical single disease control programmes and the family planning programmes'. With too much emphasis on family planning, the PHCs lost orientation and curative health delivery services were neglected. Call it lethargy or the sheer inability of the State to check these problems, the downslide further escalated in the 1980s, leading to a spurt in the private sector.[11] The mounting fiscal crisis in the country turned out to be the proverbial last nail in the coffin. Thus what necessitated health sector reforms was essentially a cumulative effect of the following: a series of unfavourable developments coupled with misguided perception of the appropriate use of health sector infrastructure as well as the inability of the State to confront with the problems emanating from several sources plus fiscal crisis. Needless to say, the 1991 economic reforms had already cleared the deck for the stated purpose. However, with the unfolding of HSR, there has been a paradigm shift wherein 'the conceptualization of health care' has changed from a 'service' to a 'commodity'[12] (for which everybody has to pay) (Priya et al., 2004: 2972).

INITIATING REFORMS: FORM, CONTENT AND PROCESS

The term 'reforms' is defined in different ways. For instance, in a broad sense, it is referred to as a paradigm shift in the delivery of (health) services. It also amounts to macro-level changes introduced in the vertically organized institutional structure. It could also be related to micro-level changes affecting any single component of the multifaceted health care services, such as health administration at the local level or improving the system of procurement and supply of drugs to the public hospitals, recruitment or deployment of health personnel in rural areas, contracting out ancillary services and so on. If we go by standard dictionary meanings, reform usually implies to improve or amend what is wrong/unsatisfactory; to change to a better state; the removal of faults or errors; to put an end to what is perceived as wrong, etc. 'The basic issue underlying any reform', says one of the foremost thinker of our time, 'is simple enough. Some existing arrangements appear to us to be not right, and we want to put them right. When dealing with public institutions or policies, the central question, then, must be: how can we improve the institutions and policies that exist and make sure that they work better?'(Sen, 2005: 1971).

In this volume, HSR is interpreted as a pronounced shift from the earlier public health policy and its impact on the functioning of public hospitals (read health care services) in the selected states. The backdrop obviously is the National Health Policy 2002. This is not to deny that the NHP 2002 has incorporated prescriptions of the World Bank underlined in its 1992 documents as it has also retained some of the key features of the (earlier) 1983 National Health Policy. For instance, the 1983 health policy admitted to encourage setting up of 'specialty and super specialty services through private investments for patients who can pay', though the justification offered for this was that 'the draw on the Government's facilities is limited to those entitled to free use' (see NHP 2002, http://mohfw.nic.in/np2002.htm p. 2). In short, the on-going process of HSR came into vogue putting strong emphasis on efficiency, efficacy and quality of health care services. This was, however, soon interpreted as an expanded role for markets. Among the multilateral agencies, the World Bank came forward offering required financing for the restructuring of intended reforms in the health sector.

Practically all states in India have adopted some form of reforms, but given their initiatives the states could be placed into two categories: the ones which have taken initiatives without any assistance from the World Bank and in the second category fall those states which have availed financial assistance. States like Gujarat, Madhya Pradesh and Tamil Nadu belong to the first category whereas Andhra Pradesh, Karnataka, Maharashtra, Orissa, Uttar Pradesh and West Bengal can be placed in the latter category. It also needs mentioning that there is an element of commonality among all these Bank-assisted states: emphasis on improving the physical infrastructure of services, particularly those related to national health sector programmes which are funded by bilateral and multilateral agencies. On the other hand, the experiences of the first category of states reveal the state-specific initiatives, confirming state autonomy allowing elbow-room for experimentation.

In a nutshell, the initiatives taken under the ongoing[13] Health Sector Reforms (HSR) comprise introduction of user fee, contracting out of ancillary services, and offering subsidies to the private sector in health services. The cause of concern, however, is the question of motivation in the implementation of the health sector reforms. This appears to be driven by the assumption that public expenditure on welfare, including curative health services, is wasteful, hence an increasing demand for a reduction in public spending and introduction of initiatives for cost recovery. Undoubtedly, this is a global phenomenon but there are variations in the extent and nature of reforms adopted by both the developed and developing countries. In addition, in many developing countries these reforms have been largely initiated under the auspices of the Structural Adjustment Programme (SAP) supported by the World Bank.

CONTEXT

Apparently, a large number of states had already taken some initiatives under the broad contours of the HSR, with or without active involvement of the international lending agencies. More than a decade had already gone by yet what was happening across the states was largely unknown. If at all some information was available, it was in bits and pieces. True, health being a state subject, therefore the matter fell largely under the domain of the state governments. But to admit that the union government had nothing much to say was travesty of truth, to say the least. To set out a national policy on the subject is decidedly the prerogative of the union government. The National Health Policy (2002) testifies to this fact. But how much of the 2002 health policy has actually been taken up and what is the state-wise status of its implementation? Set against this backdrop, a seminar on this theme was organized—'Health Sector Reforms: Public-Private Partnership and Community Initiatives'—in the fall of 2004. The objective was to capture the various strands of reforms which had started unfolding since late 1980s. Yet even at the policy level there was hardly any official document on the subject; at least not in the public domain till economic reforms started unfolding. Thus, the aim was also to utilize the opportunity to initiate debate[14] on health sector reforms.

Delivering the keynote address of the seminar, Sushma Chowdhury, the then Advisor (Health Sector), Planning Commission, stated that in the context of liberalization and privatization, the HSR weaves through various strands, though the thrust has been on Public-Private Partnership (PPP) and community initiatives. The goal in any case has been optimizing and maximizing the delivery services with key concerns for equity, quality and involvement of stakeholders. This is not to deny there is a mismatch between demand and supply, she added. For instance, on the one hand, there is absenteeism on the part of medico-personnel and on the other hand, out of 6,000 sanctioned posts under the Tenth Plan period, only 4,000 posts are filled. Besides, there is too much centralization in running the hierarchically organized health delivery services. There is a growing need for decentralization involving community, NGOs and local bodies as well as attaching due respect to diversity, and cultural flexibility in approaching the twin issues of management and quality. There are in-built lacunae in the system. Also, the reform does not seem to be addressing the system's failure. Therefore, Chowdhury emphasized, there is a need to integrate all these concerns and innovations to inform decision-making and bring about a systematic change.

Further elaborating these concerns from the perspectives of a public policy analyst, Balbir Arora (JNU) cautioned the house that 'chanting of (health) reform like a mantra' will not be of any help. It is hazy. Its 'agenda seems to be brilliantly outlined' but it does not have a roadmap. Likewise, all tall talk about the 'virtues of PPP' lacks clarity. It does talk of 'partnership' but hardly spells out the nature, scope and the terms and conditions of partnership; also, about choosing the right kind of partners. 'There is complacency about the third generation of panchayats as the action towards effective decentralization is slow and tardy'. Likewise, the 'so-called community initiatives are more akin to paternalistic/guided community support' he argued. In its utter haste to show some quantifiable, visible results, the reform process seems to be creating 'parallel, non-elective structure, bypassing cumbersome self-governing institutions.' This is a challenge which public-spirited citizenry have to squarely face. For, the need of the hour is to find ways and means to inject public service to private sector, he emphasized.

Needless to say, HSR is a complex phenomena and it comprises a host of issues. Broadly speaking it has two components: (a) internal and (b) external. The former is focussed on improving the efficiency of health care services rendered by the existing public health institutions. This includes day-to-day management of public hospitals at all the levels, supply of drugs and other consumable items, upkeep of hospital infrastructures and diagnostic instruments, skill upgradation of hospital employees, not to mention an enhanced budgetary allocation. The external component aims at expanding the health care services by forging partnership with private sector, community-based organizations as well as other local government institutions. Added to it, in both the situations is financing of health care through insurance and social security measures. An equally important issue is raising additional resources through levying user fee on patients, for smooth running of public health institutions. And if the entire exercise is rooted in the concept of efficiency and equity, as the proponents of HSR claim, naturally then it becomes crucial to look into the ideological frame of reforms and its rationale.

To bring all the interrelated issues under one cover would have been ideal but too ambitious an attempt to fructify. A modest attempt, considering the constraints, was made to focus on some, not all, of the issues concerning health sector reforms. The issues addressed in this volume are clubbed under the following sub-heads, though some of them are overlapping.

DECENTRALIZATION AND HSR

The decentralization route is one among the several accepted measures to initiate institutional reforms in the health sector. This is considered to be all the more effective towards widening the access of poor to health care services and improving its quality in the rural areas. Most importantly, decentralization is also seen as an instrument necessary to forge partnership between community-based organizations and the state institutions of health such as sub or primary health centers (NHP 2000: 9-10). The Eleventh Schedule of the Constitution that provides an inventory of functions to be devolved to PRIs categorically mentions, among others, subjects like 'health and sanitation including hospitals, primary health centre and dispensaries', 'family welfare' and 'drinking water'. The constitutional expression is absolutely clear as it intends that the PRIs should be entrusted with the 'substantial responsibility in respect of delivery of preventive, promotive and even curative health care services'. This would entail transferring of managerial responsibility to decentralized three-tiered Panchayati Raj Institutions (PRI) along with required funds and functionaries. It was indeed a bold declaration, given the vast number of such public health institutions located particularly in rural areas.

Based on the experiences of Kerala and West Bengal, two papers have discussed the impact of HSR within the broad frame of decentralization in these two states. It needs mentioning here that both these states have strong support of the cadres of the Left Front, most notably of the CPI-M, though they have followed different routes to achieve their goals. In Kerala, for instance, decentralization preceded or went along with a massive campaign for mobilizing people under the auspices of people's plan spearheaded by a voluntary organization, namely the Kerala Sahitya Praja Parishad (KSPP) which had earlier played a pioneering role in the literacy campaign. But its spread and success was largely confined to the mid-1990s when the Left Front government was in power in the state. Support of the Left Front has been equally crucial in the case of West Bengal panchayats too. In the latter case, however the continuation of the same political regime, read the Left Front, for more than a quarter of a century has turned out to be a boon. This is apparent from the fact that though the panchayats appear to be firmly rooted, nevertheless these grassroots-level institutions have been operating more like line departments or at best as extended arms of the state, than as institutions of local self-governments. Devoid of any innovation and sure of their continuation in power, largely because of a weak opposition, panchayats have been repeating what they had achieved during late 1970s and early 1980s. If strong political competition has forced the Left

Front in Kerala to innovate during their tenure, the absence of competition has made West Bengal leadership complacent in certain respects.

In the health sector, panchayats in Bengal have until recently been doing what panchayats in other states, irrespective of their life span or support of the party in power, have been engaged in. That is mobilization of people in immunization, most notably 'Pulse Polio' programme. Until recently they did not have any role to play in the day-to-day running of these sub or primary health centres[15] in the state. For long these centres had been unable to discharge their responsibilities on account of inadequate fund flow, weak infrastructure, poor supply of medicines and to cap it all absenteeism or shortage of staff. This was by and large true of health centres at the block/taluka level in most of the states, more particularly in the northern states or say barring that of Tamil Nadu, as noted earlier. If health care services were to decentralize in spirit and letter, this would necessitate transferring of managerial responsibility along with funds and functionaries to PRIs. Obviously the West Bengal government, not yet ready to undertake such a restructuring exercise, agreed to a proposal calling for a limited reform.

What is now known as the 'Amkopa experiment' discussed in detail by Ghosh (included in this volume) is of recent origin and this programme, though highly innovative and effective, has been taken up on a pilot basis. Under this scheme, women SHG members are initiated as health volunteers at the village level. The GPs are entrusted with the task of selecting the women volunteers to be trained at the PHC level. What is more remarkable about this experiment is that through this novel scheme a new awakening regarding health and hygiene has been noticed in the selected villages of Midnapur district. The women volunteers, in first place, have filled the gap left by overburdened ANMs. Secondly, villagers no longer feel helpless in case one falls sick at night, since the volunteer being local is available round the clock in the village itself. Thirdly, a comprehensive register detailing the health profile of the local people is available. Fourthly, being the facilitator and directly responsible for the performance of the volunteers (they are selected by GPs) the importance of GPs has been further enhanced. The flip side of the experiment is the reluctance of the health administration to institutionalize provision for a suitable honorarium to the lady health volunteers. In its absence, one wonders whether equally enthusiastic and committed women volunteers would come forward to shoulder this responsibility in other gram panchayats. This would also dampen the spirit of village *pradhans*, no matter howsoever enthusiastic, in due course of time.

In contrast, under the people's campaign, several initiatives were taken up in Kerala. This included additional resource mobilization and augmenting of secondary level health delivery institutions in close coordination with local self-government and PPP. Adoption of several strategies to strengthen health delivery services, the ultimate goal of HSR, in Kerala was in conjunction with decentralized planning. In any case, the reform measures taken were neither uniform nor were they implemented at the behest of the state health directorate, hence wide variations at the ground level. First of all, local people assisted by the volunteers as well as office bearers of local level institutions identified the problem and after a series of consultations arrived at a conclusion as what was feasible to realize the goal. The Nedumangad taluka (sub-district) hospital building, for instance, was in a dilapidated condition necessitating its renovation. Of course, volunteers played a key role along with the staff of the hospital but the local municipal body found a novel way to mobilize resources required for the stated purpose. It was decided to make use of the hospital land for setting up a medical shop inside the hospital. It resulted in multiple benefits. The auctioning of land fetched a substantial sum, enough for renovation and an enhanced hospital infrastructure. For patients, reliable health products were available inside the campus and that too at a cost lower than the prevailing market rates. Patients received added facilities under the same roof. All these could be realized without making any demands on the public exchequer. Doctors and support staff were happy with the added facilities that enabled them to render better services and the entire hospital ambience had improved owing to its physical uplift. Likewise under PPP a novel comprehensive community mental health care project took shape.

STATE INTERVENTION IN TAMIL NADU, ORISSA AND CHHATTISGARH

Of the state-wise experiences discussed during the seminar, the Tamil Nadu experience was quite unique as it illustrates the impact of organized state intervention having bearings on the procurement, storage and distribution of medicines to hospitals/ health centres at all the levels throughout the state. In her paper Lalitha has given a detailed account of the functioning of the Tamil Nadu Medical Service Corporation (TNMSC), an autonomous body set up as a part of reform measures adopted in the state in 1995. Till then, it needs mentioning here that like other states the procurement and distribution of medicines in Tamil Nadu was also carried out through a centralized purchasing committee. Not only was the centralized procedure cumbersome but was unable to check pilferage and wastage as well as ensuring regular supply of medicines to hospitals at all levels. In fact, the traditional system of medicine supply had given birth to many anomalies. In some health centres, for instance, there would be a stockpile of medicines that were not required, leading to wastage, whereas patients in other parts of the state would be protesting against the non-availability of the same medicines. However, in the absence of appropriate information network it was virtually impossible to correct such anomalies.

The success of TNMSC was based on the following factors: (a) an independent management board responsible for supervision and monitoring, (b) adequate financing and sound financial management, (c) public accountability, (d) transparent tendering procedure, (e) ensuring procurement of quality drugs from professionally run pharmaceutical companies. All these features are by and large common with average public sector corporations yet majority of them are not bracketed with success. What is seen to be behind the success of TNMSC is the strong pro-poor will displayed by the successive political regimes in the state. Irrespective of their nomenclature the political parties have believed in framing policies of spending more on social sectors such as health, education and nutrition than employment creation. And it has paid dividends. That TNMSC has been a success story is apparent from the fact that in the very year of its inception the corporation saved Rs. 320 million. The statistical details given in the paper also show that owing to bulk purchase by TNMSC, its per unit (medicine) prices are far lower than the prevailing market rates. Added to this was the political will of the successive regimes in the state. Besides, on an average medicines alone account for 10 to 30 per cent of total public spending on essential drugs alone.

Kundu's paper brings out Orissa-specific reforms in the health sector. First of all, it lays emphasis on the fact that HSR was prompted by an evaluation report of earlier studies of DFID and a World Bank project report on 'revamping' of secondary- and tertiary-level institutions. Like several other states, the reform process in Orissa also began with introduction of user fee at the district level but interestingly it triggered a chain of actions in other areas, too. This includes part privatization of cleaning services (with a ban on fresh recruitment of sweepers), hiring of paramedics on contract basis and also creation of a district cadre for them (largely comprising women personnel), multi-skilling of lab technicians as well as making it mandatory for medical graduates to serve in rural health centres if they wanted to enter postgraduate courses. The state health establishment has also been able to identify five major diseases responsible for morbidity and mortality and offering 'free curative treatment' to all under *Panch Byadhi Chikitsa Scheme*.

The newly created state of Chhattisgarh has also launched a community health worker programme called *mitanin*. However, unlike the Ampoka pilot project which is rooted in the community, *mitanin* is a state-sponsored scheme. Under this scheme a woman health worker is selected from the community, with self-defined hamlets rather than a village as its unit. This has been done deliberately to make the identification of the 'community' co-terminus with the gram sabha as defined under provisions of the 73rd Amendment extended in the Fifth Schedule areas. Sen's paper provides the structural arrangements of this massive state intervention and also offers a critique on this multi-layered programme. Its essential components are social mobilization along with several community-based services packages under a broad rubric of delegation and decentralization.

With the *mitanin* forming its base, the programme aims at involving both rural and urban local bodies, NGOs and hospitals. Notwithstanding the tall claims of forging multiple partnership and putting emphasis on decentralization, the fact remains that this is a highly centralized programme. Not only have the entire panchayati bodies been bypassed, rather the real power seem to have been vested in the hands of a tiny group, comprising 'ministers, bureaucrats and senior doctors' as well as a parastatal body.

INTRODUCING USER FEE

This is treated as an alternative option which a large number of states have exercised in varying degrees in the post-reform period. Yet questions are still being raised about its rationale and even its intended purpose. In first place, this strategy has been adopted to cope with the rising cost of health care and to serve evergrowing populations with depleting resources. There may have been counter-points against this provision but the fact remains that additional revenue raised through user fee serves three functions: (i) brings more autonomy in day-to-day functioning of the hospitals; (ii) results in improved infrastructure and maintenance of establishment; (iii) hospitals are able to render services all through the year (earlier centralized control of supply of consumables would result in exhaustion of X-ray films, chemicals, etc., in a few months, rendering all these services of no use during a large part of the year).

Shariff and Mondal have presented a comparative study of the impact of user fee in eight states. Although the study is based on a small sample size, it does provide us a clue to understanding its role in improving the public health care system. The states covered are: Gujarat, Karnataka, Madhya Pradesh, Orissa, Rajasthan, Tamil Nadu, Uttar Pradesh and West Bengal. The authors have shown that user charges vary even districtwise in the studied states, except in Karnataka where the charges are uniform. Interestingly, the charges are not only highest in the state of Uttar Pradesh but it is the only state where only half (50 per cent) of the entire user charges is retained at the source of collection and the rest goes to the state treasury—just contrary to the trend observed in other states. The twin issues of 'equity' and 'access of services' to poor people are addressed through the mechanism of exempting BPL category patients but its operationalization is constrained by several factors, the author duo observe. In the first place, all BPL families do not possess this particular identification card. Second, there is lack of awareness among BPL card holders regarding their entitlement (of free treatment). Finally, even if they are informed about their entitlement and own a card, they rarely carry it while visiting hospitals. For all practical purposes, therefore, identification of poor patients is largely left to the discretion of doctors, invariably chief medical officers.

The paper calls for a large survey to assess the efficacy of the provision, more particularly on issues like satisfaction of patients in general, and BPL category people in particular. Yet citing the case of Balasore Distict Hospital, the paper testifies to the positive outcome of the adopted strategy. To quote, 'Before the introduction of user fee, all equipment used to be out of order most of the time and the chief district medical officer had no power to repair those. Therefore, service was uncertain to patients. Nowadays users are also satisfied and are more confident about the hospital. Capable users are paying much less compared to private places. Patients are even ready to pay little more for better services'.

On the other hand, the authors have found several lacunae in the management and administration of this system. For instance, if all 'possible gains are not exploited', it is largely because doctors are not trained in the management of resources. Besides, what is implied in this system is that payment (of user fee) will ensure quality services. Regrettably, the health care services provided are not in tune with the expectations they have generated. If this mismatch between demand and supply is not balanced, the dissenting voices may be able to 'threaten the success of the system', the paper concludes.

The user fee also happens to be a key component of the Madhya Pradesh reforms but its impact is little different for the very simple reason that the overall reform package in this state includes other aspects. This is not to say however that the new system was performing well everywhere. Based on the functioning of the Rogi Kalyan Samiti (RKS, loosely translated as Patients Welfare Society) in the selected 10 hospitals at different levels, Kumar's study illustrates this point.

Rogi Kalyan Samiti

The RKS seeks partnership of all concerned actors at the local level to raise funds for the upkeep of the public hospitals and, in turn, ensures their participation in the management of health services. This includes participation of, administration at the local level, charitable organizations, donors, leading citizens of the area, people's elected representatives as well as hospital staff. The Madhya Pradesh HSR is all the more unique in the sense that unlike in other states, where partnership has been sought from market forces (excepting the areas where NGOs are being involved), the RKS seeks direct involvement of the users (people) and service providers (doctors, paramedicos) in running the public hospitals. Thus if the motivational factor in the case of former is profit, the latter instance is of meeting the social goals and, by extension, raising the social capital. The system as a whole has worked well in certain hospitals whereas in others it seems to have been simply dragging on. Looking at a comparative scale, the author has observed that the system suffers on three counts: first, there is a lack of information flow at the lower and even middle level of hospital staff; second, and more important, there is lack of transparency and accountability (notable exceptions apart) in the management of resources generated as also regarding outsourcing/privatization of certain services as well as recruitment of contractual staff in certain hospitals; and finally, the varying leadership attributes of the CMOs. Notwithstanding these shortcomings, if the RKS has done wonders in certain hospitals, it is largely because of the leadership quality of the hospital chief. This is all the more crucial since the new system is yet to be properly institutionalized. The paper has also noted the reversal of the system on certain counts such as attempts to narrow the support base of system, strengthening the hold of bureaucracy and politicians over the new management structure, and so on. Yet as compared to the past, the paper concludes, under the RKS the functioning of public hospitals has improved and in fact, the gains are more than visible at certain places.

PUBLIC-PRIVATE PARTNERSHIP

Described as a coping strategy or an alternative option, this has been experimented in many states in varying forms. Caught into the quagmire of shrinking budget on the one hand and growing demands for catering to the health need of the ever-increasing number of people on the other, most state governments have resorted to this option. The option is largely based on the concept of public-private partnership (PPP). The nature and extent of partnership may differ, but it is rooted in three fundamental assumptions: one, it will reduce the financial burden of the government; two, strengthen the capacity of the private sector to cater to the health needs of the people; and three, improve the quality of health care through new management structures. The well-known models of PPP (Bhatt, 2000) as practiced in most of the states (provinces) are given under: (i) offering subsidized land and exemption from excise duty on import of machinery as well as other fiscal incentives to the private sector to set up super-specialized hospitals. This model is seen in the major 18 states of the country, but they are mostly concentrated in state capitals and in a few important cities.[16] (ii) handing over management of PHCs to NGOs (e.g. Gujarat) but PHCs would continue to be wholly financed by the state government; and, (iii) involving industries in managing health centres as in Tamil Nadu. Under this scheme an industry will adopt a local primary or sub-health centre and would be responsible for building, maintaining and equipping the facility while the state government would continue providing staff and medicines.

Apart from these models of structured partnership, there are instances of other types of partnership[17] offering excellent health care to poor, particularly those who live in far flung areas. There is the model of NGOs and PHCs working in tandem to provide health care to the community. In addition to above, certain other types of partnership have been witnessed in individual states. Although not all are covered in this book, considering their uniqueness as well as their reach and impact, a few are worth mentioning.

Under this head the plan was to have two presentations: one from Gujarat and the other from Rajasthan, both representing the case of NGO-driven community initiative. But for reasons beyond our control, only the Gujarat experiment could be covered. Sewa-Rural (SR) is the NGO which pioneered comprehensive partnership with the state government to run a PHC based in Jhagadia tahsil/block of Bharuch (located between the industrially developed Surat and Vapi districts of Gujarat). It was/is an innovative 'joint venture' in more than one way, heralding a new beginning. First of all, it began in the 1980s, much before the onset of the 1991 economic reforms. Second, it opened up new possibilities: (a) the state government can be persuaded to move away from rigid thinking of 'doing all by itself'; (b) the official PHCs can be reformed from within by the deft handling of NGOs. Finally, by displaying courage and will power, SR managed to do something which until recently was unthinkable. True, SR was already engaged in areas of primary health care, therefore, it thought of experimenting by forging a partnership with the government. And to a large extent, SR was successful in realizing its goal. This is not to say that it did not face any problem with the 'partner' or even with the 'community'—the focus of its health care services. Indeed, it had to undertake trouble-shooting exercises repeatedly, following the transfer of district-level officials. The lessons SR learnt out of this unique partnership are worth documenting: persistence, patience and perseverance—the key lies in these three Ps while dealing with the government (or making the partnership workable) as well as with the community. No less important is the final outcome. Following a decade of working through a PHC, SR demonstrated that with its 'existing structure and budgetary allocations' the PHCs could still render better services with a judicious mix of decentralized decision making (particularly to reallocate budgetary heads) and planning at the local level. It also needs mentioning that through its persuasive approach it has managed to integrate the services of PHC with that of ICDS and resorted to several innovative methods for reporting, information dissemination, immunization, and referral system. Finally, the paper also underlines the imperatives of levying user fee. Among the beneficiaries of SR-piloted health care programme are a large number of poor tribals for whom the health care is absolutely free. At the same time SR arrived at the conclusion that user fee could be levied upon those who can afford to pay.

STATE, IDEOLOGY AND REFORMS

Of the two presentations on this sub-theme, Baru's paper traces the genesis of HSR and its ideological moorings. Baru has argued that the HSR is a global phenomenon and it has its roots in the neo-liberal ideology which is based on the assumption that expenditure on public systems are inefficient and therefore waste ful, hence it assigns a greater role for market forces in running efficient public delivery systems. She has attributed the ascendancy of this ideology to the two epoch-making events of preceding decades: energy crisis of the 1970s which triggered a world recession in 1980s, and later the collapse of the USSR and the east European socialist block. The failure of the world economy to deal effectively with the after-effects of these events put a question mark on the legitimacy of the role of the state in delivering collective goods to the people. The Alma Ata declaration (document on primary health, 1978) bears testimony to this fact. However, the fact remains that the public health system is already under tremendous pressure on account of the three following factors. First, the growing demand of ever increasing population; two, spiraling cost of services; and finally, the inability of the hierarchically organized health system to meet the felt needs of the people. Above all, a huge proportion of the health budget is being spent on salary and establishment alone. Thus, very little room is available to strengthen the delivery services as such. Baru's paper in a way touches upon all the core issues pertaining to reforms: its ideology and backdrop, contents of reforms, PPP, decentralization at primary and secondary level of health delivery institutions, health financing and highlights of state-wide reform initiatives.

Alain Vaguet's paper tells us the experiences of some of the European countries in the given context. In a way Vaguet seems to be complementing some of the concerns of Baru but in the European context. He also underlines the fact that HSR is a complex subject, having a number of aspects. And also that the health status of individuals in a country is directly related to the country's history, degree of development and health concern shown by its polity. No doubt, as compared to India the budgetary allocations for national health systems in the European countries are much higher. For example, it is 7 per cent of the GDP in the United Kingdom, 8.7 per cent in Sweden or for that matter 10 per cent of the GDP on health insurance in France. The system covers 85 per cent of the health expenditure of individual patients in Sweden; the corresponding figure for France is 60 per cent. In other words, 40 per cent of an individual's spending on health services is not covered under national health system in France. This in a way explains why more than 85 per cent of the French prefer to buy an additional private health insurance—a very high figure as compared to 1 per cent for Swedes and 11 per cent for British citizens. Irrespective of the system at work, however, European countries are also facing crisis mainly on two counts: rising cost of technological improvements and ageing population demanding more health attention. A strange spectacle is seen in the given context, Vaguet argues. The service providers are reluctant to reduce the cost of their services, notwithstanding the state regulation, and the elderly are afraid of the growing cost. Consequently, the reforms are not moving in the required direction.

CONCLUSION

This is a modest attempt to understand the features of HSR under implementation across the states of India. From the narratives given above, it is apparent that in most of the states the HSR are under way in varying degrees with or without the involvement of the World Bank. The international lending agency may have played a role but a close look at the form and the content of HSR suggests it to be a multi-pronged exercise designed to cope with both the fiscal and administrative/ managerial crises. In fact, some of the devices used to tide over the crises appear to be common across states. For instance, user fee has been found introduced in a large number of states. At the same time, there are state-wide variations in actual operationalization of this provision. Even in a state like Madhya Pradesh, where user fee is at the base of reforms, there are other components, including a new broad-based management structure to manage day-to-day functioning of hospitals at the local level and also oversee the use of additional resources generated. It may also be mentioned that the National Health Policy 2002 also underscores the imperative of levying user fee for certain secondary and tertiary health care services.

The experiences of West Bengal and Kerala, on the other hand, show active community involvement in furthering the cause of both reforms and decentralization, powered by 73rd and 74th Constitutional Amendments. Besides, there are unique state-wide experiences. This includes the supply of drugs in Tamil Nadu and several small but far-reaching steps being taken in Orissa to serve the poor, particularly those living in remote areas. The newly found state of Chhattisgarh is also trying to reach the poor living in remote areas, albeit through a different route. At the other spectrum of the scale, one finds equally innovative partnership forged between an NGO and the Gujarat state government. This is not to say all those listed above happen to be success stories. They are not, exceptions apart. But the successful instances give us hope for the future. And the failures also provide us with lessons to rethink the unfolding of the reforms, and the fact that a clear road map is not seen anywhere. On the contrary, even reversal has been noticed in certain cases. Yet this seems to be a larger question which cannot be viewed in isolation. For it has significant bearing on the working of the fiscal system and federalism. The former is highly centralized and the latter, with the strengthening of coalition politics and governments both at the level of states and Centre, is increasingly getting decentralized. Above all, at the level of ideology the HSR remains highly contentious. The reform process in the Western countries predates that of India but nowhere does it appear to be finally settled. Perhaps, it would never be for the very simple reason that it is an eternal quest to balance the market forces with the overarching presence of the state. Of course, it has taken a new turn since the autumn of the last century. When the governments are making endless compromises, it is too much to expect a time-bound blueprint for sectoral reforms, including health sector reforms.

POSTSCRIPT

In order to strengthen the reach and impact of health delivery services, the Government of India launched an ambitious National Rural Health Mission (NRHM) in April 2005. Its stated objective is to provide 'accessible, affordable and accountable health care' to rural population in the country. The key components of the Mission are as follows: (1) locating ASHA (Accredited Social Health Activist) in each village; (2) Health & Sanitation Committee at the level of village panchayat (VHSC) preparing village health plan; (3) invigorating rural hospitals for effective services (both curable & preventive) measurable and accountable to community; (4) minimizing inter-state and inter-district disparities; and above all (5) ensuring unmet public health needs by integrating curative health concerns with its imperatives, such as safe drinking water, nutrition and sanitation and hygiene.

Not only the NRHM accords due importance to the direct involvement of the local community represented by ASHA and VHSC but it also recognizes the fact that for the mission's success an active citizenry is *sine qua non.* No less important is inter-sectoral coordination at the district level and below. Most importantly, a cursory perusal of the above would testify to the fact that all these programmes, by and large, hinges around ASHA and VHSC, the most visible faces of the mission at the ground level, whose sincerity or slackness would make or mar prospects of the proposed initiatives.

This is important to bear in mind that the health being a state subject, the centre cannot take charge of the implementation of mission's programmes. In fact, states also lack effective control over the selection process of ASHA or formation of VHSC either. Since they are to be identified at the local level, the hold of dominant community/power takes the centre stage, it is apprehended. This becomes all the more important since the institution of gram sabha (village assembly) is yet to acquire the moral authority necessary to express the general will through wider consultations and intervene in order to ensure the common good of masses in the villages. This is notwithstanding the passage of the Constitutional (Seventy-third Amendment) Act, 1992. In fact, it was akin to misplaced enthusiasm that the prevalent caste/class/cultural divides/sub-divides in the countryside will be overcome with a legislative stroke. Thus in the absence of functional people's collectives, the powers that be in the villages (whether traditional or otherwise) would decide as who should take driver's seat (ASHA and the VHSC members in the present case) to facilitate the mission's goal at the ground level. However, the NRHM has inbuilt provision to thwart such attempts by the powerbrokers. That is, instead of paying a fixed honorarium, it provides for case based incentives to ASHA. This incentive, it is assumed, will demand promptness from ASHA, forestalling all the apprehensions regarding appropriation of ASHA by local tuff. But there is hardly any plan or time frame for meeting ambitious goals of preventive health concerns such as nutrition, public hygiene and sanitation, etc. Likewise, the mission's assurance regarding strengthening of PHCs is also vague. At another level, the role of block and district level committee are no less important in making the mission successful. Equally important is to address the frictions and contentious issues that would crop up in course of facilitating inter sectoral coordination at all the three levels: from the district to the level of village panchayat.

Several institutions of repute, besides the state-wide network of the offices under Comptroller and Accountant General, have been asked to evaluate the impact of the mission's initiatives. The evaluation reports are still awaited. But initial newspaper reports suggest that poor patients have started flocking to the public hospitals even in state like Bihar. It must be remembered that prior to unfolding of NRHM, health institutions had almost gone defunct in this state. Now with in-built incentive to ASHA for every institutional child delivery in public hospitals, there is too much rush that hospitals are finding it difficult to handle. Such teething problems may be sorted out in due course with corresponding boost in infrastructure development. Afer all, the government is pumping huge amount (Rs. 6,700 crore was its budget for 2005-6; the GOI's public spending on health has been proposed to raise from 0.9 to 2-3 per cent of India's GDP) for the success of the NRHM. But it would be naïve to believe that by scaling up budgetary allocations all the contentious issues raised above would be settled once and for all.

NOTES

1. In order to cater to the health needs of the rural populace, a three-tiered health infrastructure was laid down during the Sixth and Seventh Five-Year Plans in the 1980s. Accordingly, for a cluster of 5,000 population, a sub-centre and for every 30,000 population a Primary Health Centre (PHC) was set up. Likewise, for every 1,00,000 population a Community Health Centre (CHC) was structured. As per their organizational structure, a sub-centre is the 'peripheral contact point between the primary health care system and the community'. The PHC, in continuation, is considered to be the 'first contact point between the village community and the medical officer' but it mainly runs out-patient care, with only minimum facilities for in-patient care. Indeed, the in-patient care and treatment by specialists are available at the level of CHCs only. In plain terms, the sub-centres are run not by qualified doctors but by para-medicos known as Auxiliary Nurse Midwife (ANM). One can consult a doctor at a PHC but if a patient's condition demands continuous observation and hence admittance in the public health centre, s/he will have to go to a CHC. The available figure shows that by November 1999 a total number of 1,37,271 such sub-centres (60 per cent of which was financed by the federal government), 22,975 PHCs, and 2,935 CHCs were operating throughout the country. All these confirm huge investments in health infrastructure. But do they really provide services to the patient's satisfaction? We do not have data to confirm this point. But it is well known, 'many institutions are not fully functional due to staff shortage and non-availability of drugs and consumables. . . . Posts sanctioned in excess of norms are generally in well located PHCs to give doctors credit for rural service, aggravating the shortage in under-served areas. The problem is more serious than the vacant position indicates: the data does not capture the large-scale absenteeism of doctors in rural areas. Government doctors practice privately with or without permission, and this means inadequate attention for patients in government institutions. The overall result is the poor utilization and near collapse of the rural health infrastructure, particularly the PHCs and CHCs in most states'. See, National Sample Survey 42nd and 52nd round, Household Surveys (1991-2) of the National Council of Applied Economic Research, Delhi, cited in Misra et al., 2003: 25.

2. The Central Ministry of Health and Family Welfare comprises three independent departments: health, family welfare, and Indian Systems of Medicine (ISM). The ISM constitutes six different systems: Ayurveda, Siddha, Yoga, Unani, Naturopathy and Homeopathy. Of these only first three could be claimed as entirely indigenous. Moreover, notwithstanding a parallel infrastructure, including hospitals and teaching institutions as well as over 6 lakh registered practitioners under different streams of ISM, an overwhelming 90 per cent of incidence of illness is treated in the allopathic mode. Even registered ISM practitioners treat their patients with allopathic medicines, though they are not authorized to do so. It should also be noted that 'even though public health and family planning (FP) services had to be delivered through the common rural health infrastructure, the emphasis on FP targets have virtually transferred the entire rural health portfolio to that department, divorcing it from other health programmes'. Not surprisingly, the PHCs in many states are perceived as FP centres (Misra et al., 2003: 9).
3. It, however, deserves a mention that between 1985-6 and 1998-9, the public health spending increased by approximately 50 per cent at the primary and secondary levels whereas at the tertiary level the corresponding increase was by more than 100 per cent (ibid.: 6).
4. In short, the lack of reforms which is adding to their combined gross fiscal deficits: starting from the range of 2.40 to 2.90 per cent in 1993-4, the combined fiscal deficit of states has gone up to 4.90 per cent in 1999-2000 (Budget speech of the Finance Minister, 28 February 2001).
5. Contrast it with other Asian countries like China and Sri Lanka. Both these countries spend much lower proportion of their GDP on health (as compared to India) but their health indices are better than India's. This is largely due to the fact that the share of public health expenditure in both these countries is far greater than India's. This also explains as to why the percentage of people living below poverty line (a subsistence living below $1 per day) is much lower in China (18.80 per cent) and Sri Lanka (6.60 per cent) as compared to 44.20 per cent in India (Priya et al. 2004). The corresponding figures (the ratio of public expenditure to total health expenditure) for East Asia is 40 per cent, 50 per cent for Latin America, 75 per cent for Continental Europe and for Britain it is 85 per cent. In a way, public provisioning for health care in India is better than the following five countries in the world: Burundi, Cambodia, Myanmar, Pakistan and Sudan (WHO, 2003).
6. The private expenditure meant paying consultation fee to private doctors, purchase of medicines from the chemist shops, paying for various kinds of diagnostic tests, not to mention for admittance in private hospitals/nursing homes and so on.
7. According to the UNICEF more than a million (11.50 lakh precisely) children (below 5) in India die every year on account of malnutrition.

Ironically, one of the worst victims of this poverty-induced (malnutrition) death are children belonging to the tribal pockets of Maharashtra, otherwise considered to be a developed state in India. See, *Hindustan Times*, 15 April 2006.

8. The private health sector in India is considered to be one of the world's largest, 'with over 80 per cent of ambulatory care and 65 per cent of hospitalizations being supported through out-of-pocket expenses. Ironically the major burden of this out-of-pocket expenses is borne by those who either belong to BPL category or at best happen to live at the subsistence level, comprising nearly three-fourths of the total Indian population (Duggal, 2005: 229).
9. According to a recent survey, 'about 65 per cent of deliveries performed in the private sector end up with Caesarian, compared with 9 per cent in the public sector' (Deogaonkar, 2005). It may also be noted that in the USA, which happens to be the world's highest spender on health care (of this 40 per cent is state expenditure), nearly one-third of its population is 'denied access to basic care' (Rao, 2003).
10. Citing the 52nd Round NSS data, Duggal (2005) has also observed: '46 per cent of poorer classes and 34 per cent of the richer classes either sold assets or took loans to pay for treatment. And those using private hospitals were 16 per cent more likely to get indebted than those using public hospitals' (fn. 15: 228).
11. It may also be noted that before independence as many as three-fourth of the total doctors available in the country were in the private sector. After independence, the ideological premise of health care remained firmly rooted in patient care, serving the sick. In fact, the Bhore Committee (1946) had already underlined that it was a 'responsibility of society to ensure health care to all citizens through structures of the state. . . .' (Priya et al., 2004: 2972).
12. According to a recent estimate, the net value of the Indian health sector is 'over Rs. 1,500 billion (or US $ 34 billion). This works out to about Rs. 1,500 per capita which is 6 per cent of GDP. Of this 15 per cent is publicly financed, 4 per cent is from social insurance, 1 per cent private insurance and the remaining 80 per cent being out of personal resources as user fees (85 per cent of which goes to the private sector). Two-thirds of users are purely out-of-pocket users and 90 per cent of them are from the poorest sections' (Duggal: 229).
13. In past also some steps were taken but those being *ad hoc* remained largely ineffective. In the absence of any comprehensive planning and follow-up measures even innovative steps failed to yield desired results. In certain respects these were also a reflection of immaturity of political elites of the country. 'Barefoot doctors' scheme, based on an innovative Chinese experiment with the same caption but rooted in commune's life of 1960s, was introduced during the short interregnum of the

Janata government. This fizzled out even before it could take concrete shape, following the return of the Congress in 1980. It was retained by the Arjun Singh-led Congress government in Madhya Pradesh in 1980-5. Arjun Singh's successor and also the BJP-led state governments either ignored it or at best undermined it. With little modifications and under a different head this scheme was resurrected in mid-1990s, called Jan Swasthya Rakshak (JSR). Under this innovative scheme a youngman, educated up to 12th standard, is selected by the village panchayat, and is given training for six months during which he gets a monthly stipend. Once the training is over, he is designated as the JSR, provided with a medical kit and sent back to his village. On return, the JSR is expected to provide basic health care to villagers with the hope that users will pay him.

14. Going to the roots of the paradoxical situation, a perceptive observer had remarked: 'It is hard to think of anything more important than health for human happiness and quality of life. And yet, health is virtually absent from public debates and democratic politics in India.' This sad commentary of Jean Dreze, an economist of great repute, was based on his simple yet profound observation of 300 opinion articles published in mainstream media during the six months period (January-June 2000). To his great amazement he found none of those articles dealt with health or health-related issues. Expecting some improvement, he repeated the same exercise during the same period in 2003. This time he found a write-up on health-related issue—'it was about SARS in China'. The Tamil Nadu (along with Kerala) stands as an exception where 'health and related issues such as mid-day meals, are a subject of lively public debate and play an important role in election campaigns' (see Dreze, 2004, 'Health Checkup', *The Hindu*, 12 March 2004).

15. There were altogether 10,356, sub-centres, 922 PHCs and 346 community health centres in West Bengal, to quote 2001 census figures. Given the population-size to be covered by each of these health centres at all the three levels, there was apparently a huge gap which was to be filled up during the Tenth Plan period.

16. Among the states, concentration of such hospitals is heaviest in the four megapolis (more in Mumbai, Chennai and Delhi but less in Kolkata) and in key cities like Bangalore, Pune, Hyderabad, Chandigarh, Ahmedabad, Surat, and Vadodara. These private hospitals were in fact set up in relatively developed southern and western parts of the country. 'Those states, where private health care is prominent, have experienced either higher growth rates in agriculture incomes, as in Punjab, Haryana and Andhra Pradesh, or very high growth in demand for health care , as in Kerala', notes a data-rich study. The reverse is true in case of economically backward, poor states such

as Bihar, UP, MP, and Orissa where high levels of poverty and low incomes presumably restrict the demand for private health care' (Krishnan, 1999: 210). It may also be noted that since the 1990s, cities like Patna, and Bhubaneswar (capital city of Bihar and Orissa respectively) have also witnessed a mushrooming growth of small and medium-sized private nursing homes, signifying the near defunct status of public health institutions.

17. The Yeshasvini Health Cooperative Scheme (YHCS), for instance, covers 1.7 million farmers who happen to be members of the Karnataka Milk Federation (KMF). Under YHCS, each KMF member, mostly poor farmers and farm labourers, pays a monthly family subscription of Rs. 5. The corpus created through this subscription is managed by a trust. In return, the members get the best of health care facilities available in the state. This scheme was launched in June 2003. If the poor are unable to access heath care, it is not because of the lack of infrastructure since there is no dearth of the hospitals/nursing-homes but because of their inability to pay for the cost of the health care, says Dr. Devi Shetty, a renowned heart surgeon who pioneered YHCS for poor farmers. See, *India Today*, 17 May 2004.

REFERENCES

Baru, Rama V., *Private Health Care in India: Social Characteristics and Trends*, New Delhi: Sage, 1998.

Deogaonkar, Milind, 'Socio-economic Inequality and its Effect on Health-care Delivery in India: Inequality and Healthcare', *Electronic Journal of Sociology*, 2004, www.sociology.org/content/vol. 8.1.

Dreze, Jean, 'Health Checkup', in *The Hindu*, 12 March 2004.

Duggal, R., 'Public Health Expenditures: Investment and Financing Under the Shadow of a Growing Private Sector', in Leena V. Gangolli, Ravi Duggal and Abhay Shukla, eds., *Review of Health Care in India*, Mumbai: CEHAT, 2005.

Rao, K. Sujatha, 'Health Mustn't Hinge On Wealth', in the *Indian Express*, 24 December 2003.

David, Stephen '*Yeshasvini* Scheme: Health Without Wealth', *India Today*, 17 May 2003.

Jalan, Bimal, 'Health and Wealth', *Biblio*, March-April 2004, pp. 11-12.

Krishnan, T.N., 'Access to Health and the Burden of Treatment in India: An Inter-state Comparison', in Mohan Rao, ed., *Disinvesting in Health: The World Bank's Prescriptions for Health*, Delhi: Sage, 1999, pp. 212-30.

Ministry of Health and Family Welfare, National Health Policy 2002, http://mohfw.nic.in/np2002.htm

Misra, Rajiv et al., *India Health Report*, New Delhi: OUP, 2003.

Nandraj, S., V.R. Muraleedharan, Rama Baru, Imrana Qadeer, and Ritu Priya, *Private Health Sectors in India: Review and Annotated Bibliography, Chennai*: IIT, New Delhi: JNU, 2001.

Priya, Ritu, Alpana Sagar, Rajib Dasgupta, Sanghamitra Acharya, 'CMP on Health: Making India World Class', *Economic and Political Weekly*, 3 July 2004, pp. 2971-4.

Qadeer, Imrana, 'The World Development Report 1993: The Brave New World of Primary Health Care', in M. Rao, ed., *Disinvesting in Health: The World Bank's Prescriptions for Health*, 1999, pp. 49-64.

Rao, M. (ed.), *Disinvesting in Health: The World Bank's Prescriptions for Health*, Delhi: Sage, 1999.

Sankar, D. and Vanish Kathuria, 'Health System Performance in Rural India: Efficiency Estimates Across States', *EPW*, 27 March 2004, pp. 1427-33.

World Bank, *World Development Report*, New Delhi: OUP, 1993.

CHAPTER 2

Decentralizing Health Care Delivery System in West Bengal: A Review of the Recent Initiatives

BUDDHADEB GHOSH

The Department of Health and Family Welfare (DHFW) of West Bengal has, in the recent years, initiated several measures for reforming the health sector. Among them, decentralization of the health and medical care delivery system is claimed to be one. In its document on 'Health Sector Strategy 2004-2013', the department identifies four overall objectives of the reform, two of which are as follows:[1]

- To improve the accessibility of poor and unreached groups to curative, preventive, promotive and rehabilitative health services;
- To ensure quality at all levels of health and medical care services.

The need for decentralization arises from the concern for achieving these two important objectives. It has also been felt that decentralization of the delivery system would create enabling conditions for the Community-Based Organizations (CBO) to enter into partnership with state institutions in providing health care, which, in turn, would facilitate wider accessibility of the primary health services.

DECENTRALIZATION INITIATIVES

Improving the accessibility of the primary health care facilities, particularly the improved accessibility of the poor and the unreached groups of the rural areas, depends principally upon the spread of and the quality of services available at the sub-centres, Primary Health Centres (PHC) and the Block Primary Health Centres (BPHC). There are at present 10,356 sub-centres, 922 PHCs and 1146 BPHCs in the state to quote 2001 census as against the requirement of 13,611 sub-centres, 2,263 PHCs and 567 BPHCs as per the 1991 census. Clearly there is a big gap in so far as the spread of the health care facilities in the rural areas are concerned, part of which is likely to be filled up during the Tenth Five-Year Plan Period.

In the present paper, we are not concerned with the problem of adequate coverage of the health and medical care facilities. Our focus is on improving the quality of services available at the existing institutions and on the accessibility of the rural people, especially the poor and the unreached among them, to such services. The policy of the state government also is to give priority to the strengthening of the existing institutions, rather than proliferating substandard health centres. As the above figures reveal, the number of the health and medi-care facilities already created in the rural areas of the state is quite formidable. That they cannot be managed centrally is too obvious an observation to need further elaboration. Yet, this was precisely the case till the health sector reform of the state started in the beginning of the present decade. Under the traditional system, the local-level officials had little powers to take managerial and financial decisions and there was too much bureaucratic control from above. The involvement of the panchayati raj institutions (PRIs) in the management of the health institutions at the district and sub-district levels was non-existent. Consequently, there was little transparency in the health sector activities and the accountability of the health officials to the local people or to their representatives was conspicuous by its absence.

It is a common knowledge that the quality of the services available at the medi-care institutions of the state in the rural areas leaves much to be desired. Mass media quite often bring out stories of malfunctioning of the health care centres in the villages. Complaints are frequently made about the poor infrastructure of the health centres, shortage or indiscipline of medical or para-medical staff, poor supply of medicines and the like. Without disregarding the importance of the issue of inadequate fund flow that stands at the root of many weaknesses of the existing facilities, it cannot be denied that centralized and bureaucratic control over the grassroots-level health institutions was acting as a major constraint in optimizing benefits from them.

In view of the above, one of the early reform initiatives related to the decentralization of decision-making powers in respect of day-to-day management of the health and medical care institutions at the district and the sub-district levels. For this purpose the state government has created a District Health and Family Welfare Samiti (DHFWS) at the district level and a Block Health and Family Welfare Samiti (BHFWS) at the block level. Both these samitis are registered bodies and their governing bodies are headed by the chairpersons of zilla parishad and panchayat samiti respectively. Chairpersons of the standing committees on health of the respective levels of panchayat are represented in the district and block samitis' governing bodies. Chief Medical Officer of Health (CMOH) of the district is the member-secretary of the district-level samiti. Similarly the Block Medical Officer of Health (BMOH) is the member-secretary of the block-level samiti. MLAs of the district—one each from all the political parties—and representatives of the NGOs operating in the district are also members of the district samiti. The district Magistrate is the Executive Vice-Chairperson of the district samiti. In the block samiti, BDO along with some representatives from the gram panchayat are represented in the governing bodies.

The governing bodies of the samitis have to meet at least once in three months. For taking routine managerial decisions, there is an Executive Committee at the district level, which is headed by the District Magistrate (DM) in his capacity as Executive Vice-Chairperson of the district samiti. The financial powers of CMOH have been enhanced considerably.

The DHFWS has been given substantial administrative and financial powers. These include routine maintenance of equipment, procurement and distribution of medicines and medical stores, imposing and recovering fees and charges for providing services, subject to the guidelines of the government in this regard. They also can receive and utilize donations and funds from various donor agencies without the requirement of depositing the same in the government treasury. Powers to transfer the medical and other health department staff within the district have also been given to the samiti, thus facilitating proper utilization of available staff in different medical care institutions. Previously, much of such powers belonged to the directorate or to the department.

DECENTRALIZATION OR DECONCENTRATION?

A centralized health delivery system has many pitfalls. Decentralization, it is argued, is essential to make the delivery system relatively more efficient and cost effective. It is also advocated for the purpose of making the system transparent and accountable to the local people. Various policy papers of the central government including the National Health Policy have promoted decentralization. What is of more significance is that the direction to decentralize the rural health delivery system finds place in the Constitution of the country. The Eleventh Schedule of the Constitution, which provides the list of functions or activities fit for being devolved to the panchayati raj bodies, specifically mentions, among others, items like 'health and sanitation including hospitals, primary health centre and dispensaries', 'family welfare' and 'drinking water'. This demonstrates clearly the constitutional intention of sharing the state's responsibility of providing health care services with the PRIs. The responsibility that is proposed to be given to the panchayats is by no means nominal, as this includes also the management of the public sector hospitals and health centres in the rural areas. In other words, the Constitution expresses the intention that the PRIs should shoulder substantial responsibility in respect of the delivery of preventive, promotive and even curative health care services. This includes management of the sub-centres, PHCs, BPHCs and similar kinds of small indoor or outdoor health care facilities. Considering the number of such public sector facilities required for the rural areas, this is, no doubt, a very sensible and bold direction.

In its various policy statements, the DHFW argues in favour of decentralization and involvement of the PRIs in delivering health services in the rural areas. It is claimed that the decision has been taken to decentralize the 'sector governance through involvement of PRIs in planning, implementing, monitoring and evaluating health, family welfare, nutrition and sanitation services in rural areas'.[2] According to another policy statement, one of the strategies of the state government 'to improve the accountability, transparency, coverage, equity and quality of health services' is to 'develop partnerships with panchayati raj institutions'.[3]

Despite such unequivocal statements, the route followed by the West Bengal government in respect of decentralization of the health sector marks a departure from the one prescribed in the Constitution. 'Partnership with' or 'involvement of' PRIs for the delivery of health services may begin only after devolution of powers and responsibilities to them. In concrete terms this would mean transfer of the grassroots-level institutions (such as, sub-centres, PHCs, BPHCs), staff attached to them and funds to the PRIs. It is difficult to understand how the PRIs are expected to get involved in 'planning, implementing, monitoring and evaluating' the health programmes without similar kind of devolution of institutions, staff and funds. One may recall that this is the route that the state of Kerala followed when it decentralized the health delivery system, along with other grassroots-level functions, under the 'People's Plan Programme' in the mid-1990s.

What West Bengal has done is in the nature of de-concentration whereby the decision-making powers of the field-level officers of the health department have been enhanced. This was, no doubt, an appropriate decision and it is claimed that it is yielding good results.[4] But the fact remains that this is no more than a managerial reform and it can ultimately have very limited results. What the situation demands and what the Constitution envisages is a systemic reform. The systemic ills cannot be cured by managerial reforms alone. Under the present system 'accountability continues to flow along vertical lines'. Without accountability to the local government institutions, the present arrangement is unlikely to improve significantly the 'transparency in operations'.[5]

The establishment of registered societies at the district and block levels creates, in reality, an illusion of decentralization. Placing chairpersons of the zilla parishad and panchayat samiti at the head of these societies and nominating some NGO representatives in their governing bodies do not make them popular and representative bodies. They are like other bureaucratic committees created and run by the state government. In fact, predecessor to the district health and family welfare society was a district level committee with more or less the same membership. The only innovation brought by the reform was to replace a number of such committees by one committee. This committee has now been converted into a registered society at the district level. The other innovation was to set up first a committee and then a registered society at the block level. The state-sponsored societies are for all practical purposes parts of the state government. They may be allowed either to develop as full-fledged parastatal organizations like District Rural Development Agency, Fish Farmer Development Agency, SC and ST Development Corporation and so on, or they may serve as mere committees without disturbing the basic organizational features of the existing field units of the state government. In the former case the activities are run in the name of the parastatal organizations, while in the second case not even this semblance of autonomy is granted. It is the second pattern that has been adopted in respect of the district-level and block-level societies for health and family welfare. Such an arrangement may be euphemistically called decentralization, but, in effect, it is nothing more than a case of deconcentration. Similarly, association of the chairpersons or other members of the panchayati raj bodies in the governing bodies of the registered societies does not amount to the involvement of such bodies in the management of the health programmes.

When the health sector reform started back in 2001, one of the measures was to designate the health assistants attached to the sub-centres as ex-officio gram panchayat health assistants. They were expected to work under the supervision of the gram panchayats. This was a correct step towards decentralization. But this line appears to have been abandoned or, at least, postponed in the later period. The later orders on the sub-centres speak a lot about their reorganization and gram panchayat's responsibility in planning and running the sub-centre activities, but prefer to remain silent on the transfer of institutions, staff or funds to the panchayats. Moreover, the panchayats have not yet been given responsibility to run the *Anganwadi* centres, which have a useful role to play in providing health care services especially for children and their mothers. Being run by another line department, namely Department of Women and Child Development, these centres work independently of both the PRIs and the sub-centres or PHCs, which are run by DHFW. The much-needed field-level coordination between the two delivery systems could have been facilitated by devolving managerial responsibilities of these grassroots-level organizations to the PRIs. By avoiding the issue of devolution of powers and responsibilities in respect of local-level health care services to the local government institutions, the possibilities of building an institutional framework for field-level coordination between different delivery systems for achieving the same objectives are being unnecessarily sacrificed. Thus the decentralization initiatives of West Bengal's health department show signs of ambivalence. The need for active involvement of PRIs is recognized, but the government is reluctant to give up its direct managerial control over the grassroots-level health institutions. At the same time, the government also seeks panchayat's cooperation in running them efficiently. Thus the registered societies come into being as a kind of a 'compromise formula' of carrying out basically the 'agenda of deconcentration and not devolution'.[6]

FROM DECONCENTRATION TO DEVOLUTION: INCREMENTAL PROGRESS?

In October 2004, the state government introduced some changes in the administrative arrangements for monitoring, supervising and reporting of the rural health care services. In the changed system, the three-tier PRIs have been brought closer to the grassroots level health care institutions like sub-centres, PHCs and *Anganwadi* centres. Henceforth, the gram panchayats and the panchayat samitis would be involved in planning, monitoring and delivery of promotive and preventive health care services in collaboration with the line department officials attached to the above institutions. At present such involvement is more substantive in respect of monitoring of the services. For this purpose, it has been decided that the health officials, namely the health assistants and health supervisors, will have to present reports on field situation in the monthly meetings of the standing committees of gram panchayat and panchayat samiti dealing with health-related matters. Besides, they would work in close collaboration with the panchayats. In respect of planning and implementation of programmes for improving the reach and the quality of the services, panchayats will play a facilitative, rather than an implementative role. The latter still belongs to the field organizations of DHFW. But with the authority to monitor the field situation on a regular basis, the panchayats are expected to exert their influence on the functioning of the field organizations of the line department. If not anything else, this is likely to ensure that the field-level health officials remain accountable not only to their departmental superiors but also to the local panchayats.

The specific areas in which the PRIs will focus their attention are as follows:

- Collection of detailed information about and ensuring registration of births and deaths
- Safe motherhood, including prevention of marriage before 18 years in the case of female and 21 years in respect of male persons
- Family planning
- Prevention of malnutrition of children, especially of those in the age group of 0-3 years
- Infrastructure of sub-centres, PHCs and *Anganwadi* centres
- Supply of safe drinking water
- Sanitation and personal hygiene

In the case of the last two items, panchayats already have direct responsibility. Henceforth such responsibility will assume greater importance in view of the role given to them for delivery of preventive health care services.

Earlier, panchayats did not have any responsibility in respect of development or maintenance of the infrastructure of the grassroots-level health care centres. Under the new dispensation, the gram panchayat and panchayat samiti have to play a big role in this area. In an order issued in May 2005, the DHFW has transferred management of all immovable assets like land

and structures including electrical and sanitary fittings and other facilities to the panchayat samiti in respect of the BPHC and PHCs and to the gram panchayat in respect of sub-centres. Funds for this will be provided by the DHFW. Additionally, the PRIs will be entitled to use their own funds for the same. They have been given full powers to execute works for improvement of the physical infrastructure of the health institutions. However, for construction of new structures they have to obtain prior approval of the DHFW. Traditionally the Public Works Department (PWD) used to discharge the responsibility of management of the physical assets of all public institutions including those of the health centres at the block or village levels. By transferring the function relating to the maintenance and improvement of land and structures of BPHC, PHCs and the sub-centres from PWD to the PRIs an important step has been taken toward devolution. The gram panchayats have also been given jurisdiction in improving the physical facilities of the *Anganwadi* centres for which they have been authorized to utilize the untied as well as SGRY funds. All these are likely to make an impact upon the quality of health care services at the grassroots level.

The latest decisions have three important features, which should be noted. First, the panchayats have been empowered to influence the functioning of the PHCs and sub-centres in respect of promotive and preventive health care services. This has been ensured without making any radical change in the authority-structure of the DHFW. The only change introduced is that panchayats have been authorized to monitor the status of public health in the local areas and to plan and implement activities in collaboration with the line department for improving the reach and the quality of health care services. This may make the field officials of DHFW a little more transparent and accountable to the local government institutions. Secondly, for the first time the panchayats have been given some responsibility in delivering health care services. This is likely to open up new possibilities, because institutional framework for introducing local-level participatory planning in the delivery of health care services will be available and given the involvement of panchayats, opportunities for community participation and augmentation of resources for health care will be brighter. Additionally, the DHFW will find an effective facilitator at the field level in discharging its responsibility of providing promotive and preventive health care services in far-flung villages. Thirdly, by transferring the very important function of maintaining the physical assets of the local-level health institutions from PWD to the panchayats, an important step has been taken toward devolution.

West Bengal thus presents an interesting example of the tortuous process of systemic reform in the public sector. Decentralization had been accepted for quite some time as a major institutional reform necessary for improving the quality of and widening access to the health care services in the rural areas. This called for transfer of managerial responsibility of the grassroots-level health care institutions together with staff and funds to the PRIs. Yet, the state government went for deconcentration type of decentralization, while recognizing at the same time the need for the assumption of responsibility by the panchayats in the delivery of health services in the rural areas. As described above, through its latest policy decisions the state government has moved forward from its rather conservative and ambivalent approach toward decentralization. Does this signal an intention to go for full-scale decentralization of rural health care delivery system in an incremental way? One has to wait for some time to get a categorical answer to this question.

COMMUNITY PARTICIPATION

It is being increasingly recognized that Community-Based Organizations (CBO) have an important role to play in improving the outreach and the quality of the health services in the rural areas. For, the rural health system institutions have their own limitations, which cannot be overcome without community participation. It is worthwhile to identify them in order to appreciate the necessity of community initiatives in improving the outreach of health care facilities.

First, there is lack of awareness about preventive health care practices among many villagers, particularly among the poor. The health workers and the ANM are there to spread the required information. But they have to attend the sub-centre clinics thrice a week and find little time to visit individual households of about five or six thousand people. Second, people in remote villages feel helpless when immediate assistance is needed, particularly during the night. The health officials of the sub-centres or the PHCs do not generally live in the local areas, commuting to their work places from the nearby towns. Distance from the hospital coupled with the lack of transportation facilities and, sometimes, lack of awareness lead people quite often to the quacks or faith healers, thus endangering the lives of patients. Third, despite the existence of the facilities, prenatal and postnatal care of women are often neglected. Pregnancies are often not reported on time. A strong need is felt to motivate pregnant women to take appropriate care before, during and after childbirth. Fourth, information about the outbreak of a disease in a remote area does not often reach the sub-centres or health centres promptly, thanks to the lack of an institutional arrangement for communication between the villagers and the service providers. Fifth, there exist in the remote rural areas many social prejudices, practices and superstitions, which cause adverse effect upon community health. Mobilizing public opinion against them has also to be a part of the programme aimed at improving the health status of the community. Last but not the least, there is a necessity of providing a linkage and facilitating interactions between the community and the providers of various services needed for improving the health status of people. They include not only health system institutions, but also institutions like *Anganwadi* centres, and primary schools to access the services available for children and the panchayats to ensure facilities like sanitation, drinking water, midday meals for school-going children and the like.

It is difficult for the state institutions to address these issues. But village-based CBOs may play a useful role in addressing them and in discharging, in the process, certain essential functions for which there exists an institutional gap. In the discourse on development, it is often forgotten that in certain sectors, interventions become necessary at the micro level. Health of the rural communities is one such sector where development interventions need to be undertaken on a regular basis, not once in a while, to the individual households, neighbourhoods or village communities. It is not possible for any state institution, or even the panchayats, to expand in a manner that could enable them to make micro interventions of such kind. Hence the need for a community-based institution, which in collaboration with the health system institutions and the local panchayat, can undertake such tasks. Examples of the health related functions that such an organisation may possibly discharge in partnership with the state institutions and the panchayats are indicated in Table 2.1.[7]

TABLE 2.1: ROLE OF THE CSOs IN HEALTH-RELATED FUNCTIONS

Functions	*Some examples of the role of the CSOs*
Providing services	• First-aid, emergency management of simple ailments, such as diarrhoea. • Distributing essential medicines, condoms, bleaching powder, materials for constructing sanitary latrines, etc., and so on. • Facilitating community interaction with the panchayat and health institutions like the sub-centre, and health centre. • Organizing immunization and health camps. • Supporting the health workers. • Arranging training of the local midwife.
Preventive and promotive activities	• Disseminating health information. • Promoting personal hygiene practices, especially for children. • Campaign for changing social attitudes which are harmful for women and girl children.
Equity	• Promoting and facilitating pro-poor activities for enabling the unreached to access health services. • Mobilizing public opinion in favour of pro-poor policies.
Resource mobilization	• Generating local resources to provide health services.
Monitoring	• Monitoring the quality of health services. • Channelizing complaints and claims.

THE CBO AND COMMUNITY HEALTH: EMERGING POSSIBILITIES

CSOs in West Bengal are not strong. NGOs are present in many areas, but excepting a handful of them, none is strong enough to create big impact, especially in the health sector. Strong movements for creating community-based institutions are also conspicuous by their absence. Accordingly a viable model for state-community partnership to improve the health status of rural people did not grow. In recent years, possibilities for the same are opening up, thanks to local initiatives in some districts. It will be rewarding to take note of these initiatives, especially the one of Amkopa Gram Panchayat of Garbeta I Block of Paschim Medinipur district where the idea of *swasthya sahayika*—the village-based voluntary health worker—was born and given shape and then replicated in 19 other gram panchayats of the district. Though barely two-years old, the idea of voluntary health workers drawn from the self-help groups of women has attracted much attention. M.S. Swaminathan feels that '*swasthya sahayikas* can become catalysts of a health revolution in rural India' and he proposes to incorporate the 'remarkable experience of Paschim Medinipur' in his 'bio-village paradigm of human centred development'.[8]

THE AMKOPA EXPERIMENT

On a hot day in May 2003, the DM of Paschim Medinipur was visiting the on-going work of tank excavation in Amkopa Gram Panchayat of Garbeta I Block. As it happens during such visits, the *pradhan* (chairperson) of the local gram panchayat along with other local leaders utilized this opportunity to discuss various local problems with the DM. One of the problems that found prominence in that day's discussion related to the health care. There are three sub-centres in the gram panchayat area, which has a population of 19,000. The *pradhan* and the local people were demanding another sub-centre for the area to which they were entitled according to the norm of one sub-centre per 5,000 people. They pointed out that the load on the existing centres was quite high and the health officials attached to the centres were finding it very difficult to provide satisfactory services. In the discussions that followed on that afternoon, it became apparent that given the state's resources, sanction of another sub-centre in a GP where already three such centres exist, was not possible in near future. Besides, it became clear that for improving the outreach of health services, villagers needed the services of multi-purpose health workers more intensively and, as such, it would be ideal to have such workers in every village. This need could not be met by opening up another sub-centre. Self-help initiatives of the community could, on the other hand, remove many difficulties the villagers were facing in accessing health care services. This kind of thinking gave birth to the idea of drawing voluntary health workers from the Self-Help Groups (SHG) of the villages. Fortunately, quite a large number of self-help groups were functioning in the area and the rural women were showing considerable interest in the various saving and income generating activities of such groups.

The idea of involving the SHGs in the health delivery system and identifying voluntary health workers or *swasthya sahayikas* from among their members caught the imagination of the officials, the *pradhan* of the gram panchayat and the local political leadership. They saw in it a possibility of offering some essential health-related services to the people of distant villages. Within a short time the local panchayat and other leaders identified around 40 women from the various SHGs to serve the people of over 30 villages/neighbourhoods of the gram panchayat. The criteria of selection were threefold: first, they should be residents of the village to be served by them; second, they should agree to serve on voluntary basis; third, they should have read at least up to standard VIII.

After selection, the prospective *sahayikas* were called for a meeting, which was also attended by the officials, including the Block Medical Officer, and the panchayat representatives. Their role was briefly outlined and they were asked to start the work of a health status survey of every household in the prescribed format to elicit information on such matters as the nature of ailments and their treatment together with medical expenses incurred in the last one year, pregnancy, child birth, adoption of family welfare methods, nutrition, sanitation and drinking water facilities, immunization status, personal hygiene practices, etc. After they started the survey work, a formal training course was arranged for them and this included practical demonstration in the block primary health centre. Some of the aspects covered in the training were as under:[9]

- Immunization schedule of pregnant women and children;
- Nutrition of mother and the child;
- Diarrhoea management;
- First-aid for snake bite, cuts, burns and other injuries;
- Personal hygiene practices including sanitation and handling of drinking water;
- Family welfare methods and options;
- Preparation of low-cost baby food.

After training, the *sahayikas* were provided with a medical kit containing essential items like first-aid equipment and materials, ORS packets, common medicines, antibiotic ointment, thermometer and bleaching powder. They were also provided with cycles.

The first thing the *sahayikas* of Amkopa did was to visit every household under their charge to collect health data. Roughly every *sahayika* has under her charge 60 to 100 households. They started advising the household members directly on various preventive health care matters. In order to look credible, they themselves started following hygienic practices in their personal lives. For example, the *sahayika* got sanitary toilets constructed in their houses before they started advising people on sanitation. It took some time before they could earn some credibility. Their credibility increased when they could provide some concrete services that included providing assistance to people to access the facilities available at the local health system institutions. Their direct interaction with the sub-centre staff and, in some cases, with the doctors of the PHCs enabled the *sahayikas* to bridge the missing link between the community and the health system institutions. It may be worthwhile to share some of the specific experiences of the *sahayikas* of Amkopa and Garanga Gram Panchayats of Garbeta I Block.

Hira Maity of village Nepura says: 'At present many women come to my house to ask remedy for small problems like cuts, wounds, fever and children's diseases. I give them some common medicines and advise them to go to a hospital or sub-centre if the problem so demands. I took initiative for vaccination of pregnant mothers and for meeting their nutrition needs'.

Renuka Kundu of village Lakhanpur says: '(Among other things,) I advised women to wash their utensils in clean water (and not in the unclean water of the village pond). They followed my suggestion and the problem of (water-borne diseases) is diminishing. . . . I gave iron tablets to pregnant mothers and prepared diet charts for them. . . . (After I joined) I could motivate at least 12 households to construct sanitary latrines. I am trying hard to ensure that every house has one sanitary latrine'.

Jharna Roy of Kharkata colony says: 'I gave ORS to 10 patients . . . and I sent 30 persons who were suffering from fever to the sub-centre. One of them was found to be suffering from malaria. He was sent to the hospital and he recovered. . . . There were seven pregnant women. I talked individually to each of them and gave proper advice. . . . I disinfected 18 wells of the village by spreading bleaching powder.'[10]

Bandana Maity of Garanga gram panchayat says: 'Once a child got injured in the head. I gave first-aid and some emergency medicines. Then I persuaded the mother to take the child to the hospital'.

Both Hasinara of Garanga GP and Hira Maity of Amkopa GP say: 'Sometimes we are called even in the midnight to tackle a patient. We give appropriate advice for treatment and also supply emergency medicines, if necessary. In extreme cases, we help the households to take the patient immediately to the hospital.'

Dipti Mandal, ANM attached to a sub-centre of Amkopa GP informed that after the *sahayikas* started their work, she could notice visible improvement in certain areas. For example, information about outbreak of diseases in remote villages was coming much faster than before; registration of pregnant mothers and their check-ups had increased significantly and awareness about immunization of children was increasing.[11]

Examples of such varied experiences may be multiplied, but this is not necessary. Even the few examples provided here show that the idea of having one *swasthya sahayika* drawn from the local CBO (self-help group in the present case) for every village or for 100 households or so in a village was a very simple but an important innovation. For, the *sahayikas* were bridging a missing link between the community and the rural health system.

FROM EXPERIMENT TO POLICY: PARTNERSHIP WITH THE PANCHAYAT AND THE COMMUNITY

The experiences of Paschim Medinipur led the West Bengal government to introduce in the whole state a system of health care management that would require the state's grass-roots level health institutions to enter into a partnership with the gram panchayat and the self-help groups. Government orders in this respect were issued towards the end of 2003. The main features of the policy of involving the gram panchayat and self-help groups in health care management are as follows.

- The sub-centres will be reorganized in consultation with the standing committees on health of the gram panchayat, panchayat samiti and zilla parishad.
- One of the sub-centres within a gram panchayat will be located in the village where the panchayat office is located. Preferably, it will be housed within the panchayat office building or at a place adjacent to it. This will be designated as headquarters sub-centre. This centre will be adequately staffed with one superviser and health assistants. The headquarters sub-centre will supervise and coordinate the works of other sub-centres within the GP.
- The self-help groups in different villages will be involved in health care management more or less in the pattern developed in Amkopa and other GPs of West Medinipur.
- The role of gram panchayat will be as follows:
  - To take responsibility of preventive and promotive health care measures and to provide assistance for curative health care.

- To select the self-help group and one volunteer from each such group to serve roughly 100 households in each village/ neighbourhood.
- To collect health-related data through the volunteers of self-help groups and prepare a health plan for the panchayat area.
- To take initiative for training of the *sahayika* or health volunteers and to coordinate their activities.
- To coordinate the functioning of the sub-centres and to ensure that an effective linkage is established between them and the self-help groups/health volunteers.
- To ensure that the health sub-centres supplement the activities of ICDS centres, especially in respect of immunization of children.

Sustainability of the Policy

The model described above was to be launched in the beginning of 2004. Each zilla parishad was requested to launch the model initially in those gram panchayats where the self-help groups had made some progress. To provide direction to the new initiative of involving the communities and gram panchayats in the health delivery system, special cells had been created with qualified medical officers in each zilla parishad and at the department of panchayat and rural development. But the progress in this regard has been tardy. It seems that the state government itself is not quite confident about the feasibility of the idea of drawing voluntary health workers from the self-help groups. Yet, as demonstrated in Paschim Medinipur district, it is a useful innovation and has the strength of fulfilling an institutional gap that exists at present. But there are valid reasons to believe that in the present form, its institutionalization and sustainability are doubtful.

In the first place, the process of transferring the responsibility of health care management to the panchayats and endowing them with commensurate powers and resources is not yet complete. As noted already, in respect of devolution, the government is proceeding in a very cautious, if not in a somewhat ambivalent, manner. For ensuring community participation, initiatives of panchayats are necessary. In the absence of devolution, panchayats may not have either enough motivation or the power to discharge effectively various responsibilities given to it, namely, health planning, establishing linkages between the SHGs and the health institutions, supervision and co-ordination of various kinds of health activities in the area. Even though some powers have been given to the PRIs recently, more needs to be done in respect of full-scale decentralization. It is believed that community participation is dependent upon initiatives taken by the local leadership, which, in turn, depend upon the vibrancy of local democracy. Devolution-type of de-centralization assumes importance in this context.

Secondly, the model rests in a large measure upon the voluntary health worker, so far as community participation is concerned. Such an arrangement has its limitations, because the *sahayikas* cannot be expected to render voluntary service endlessly. It is argued that being a member of the SHG, the *sahayika* has some opportunity to earn income and, accordingly, she may not deny giving voluntary service for community health care. This argument does not hold good. For, exceptional people may be there, but to find them in every village will be too ambitious. Some expectation of financial incentive, even if it is a pittance, seems natural, if the *sahayika* has to render service continuously and efficiently.

Thirdly, there is a necessity to raise local resources to improve the local-level public health and medi-care services. Local resource generation is necessary not only for paying small honoraria to the *sahayikas*, but also for ensuring continuous supply of medicines or equipment. Flow of health department's funds is unlikely to be either timely or sufficient. Accordingly it is necessary to build a corpus of funds at the community and panchayat levels by taking regular contributions (say Rs. 10 per month per household) from the villagers. Even if poor families are left out, there will remain at least 50 to 60 per cent of households in most of the villages who may agree to contribute, provided they get quality and prompt services from the *sahayikas* and health institutions. A part of such fund may be utilized for paying honoraria to the *sahayikas*, and the rest for buying medicines and equipment. In the present policy framework, there is a vague recognition of the fact that the *sahayikas* deserve some small honoraria, which may be realized by taking contributions from the rural households. But the whole issue of raising local resources not only to pay the *sahayikas*, but also to meet other expenses does not receive adequate attention.

It is not difficult to overcome these deficiencies and, hence, it is also possible to institutionalize a model that would ensure partnership of SHGs, panchayats and the state's health system institutions in the delivery of health care services in the villages. Unfortunately, the state government still seems to be in search of a viable model for community participation.

CONCLUSION

The underlying premise of the paper is that 'political decentralization' and 'civic decentralization' are essential for improving the services of the grassroots-level health care institutions and for ensuring wide accessibility of the rural households to the various health care services. 'Political decentralization' refers to the empowerment of panchayats through devolution of responsibility, powers and resources to them and 'civic decentralization' refers to the space given to the community participation in the delivery of services. It has been shown that both political and civic decentralization constitute an important part of West Bengal's health sector reform policy also. But, as this paper argues, progress in this respect has been unsatisfactory. The state government took hesitant steps towards devolution, opting initially to go for only deconcentration. Even though the government has taken some steps towards devolution recently, much remains still undone. The state has also so far failed to achieve success in scaling up implementation of any viable model of community participation. Nevertheless the state does not seem to have abandoned the idea that a systemic change in the form of political and civic decentralization of the health care delivery system is necessary for improving the quality of and widening the access to health care services in the rural areas. Largely because of this, the West Bengal story is of some value to others.

NOTES

* The author acknowledges with gratitude the support received from Dilip Ghosh, Biswajit Ghosh, Niranjan Sarkar, Bansibadan Mandal, Jiten Dey, *pradhans*, *sahayikas* and the health staff of Amkopa and Garanga gram panchayats in preparing this paper. They are, however, not responsible for any errors, omissions or views.

1. www.wbhealth.gov.in
2. 'Health Strategy Document 4: Integrated Financial and Economic Plan of the Health Sector', www.wbhealth.gov.in
3. 'The Health Sector Strategy 2004-2013', www.wbhealth.gov.in
4. Health Minister's budget speech, 2003.
5. 'Health Strategy Document 3: Overview of DHFW Activities', www.wbhealth.gov.in
6. Ibid.
7. Adapted from 'Health Strategy Document' 3.
8. 'Introduction', in M.V. Rao, *Community Health in Community Hands*, Medinipur: Mithu Enterprise, 2003.
9. Rao (2003).
10. Ibid.
11. Author's interview with the *sahayikas* and the health staff on 9 August 2004.

CHAPTER 3

Health Sector Reforms in Kerala: Decentralization Initiatives and the Lessons

JOY ELAMON

INTRODUCTION

Health sector reforms have become a major concern around the world today. Decentralization is one of the key elements in health system reforms. There are arguments that decentralization promises more direct accountability of public health and health care institutions, more efficient management of resources, better linkages between information and planning, easier inter-agency coordination and the ability to respond effectively to the variety of different needs and capacities of different regions and localities.[1]

One of the three forms of decentralization—deconcentration, delegation and devolution—is being chosen to attempt to solve particular problems. Chile deconcentrated a few of the public health services to 27 autonomous health service areas, while devolving health care services to 325 municipalities. Kenya devolved cost-sharing authority to District Health Management Boards in the 1980s.[2] Indonesia experimented with deconcentrated data gathering and related planning of some health programmes to provincial health offices in three provinces in the 1980s and expanded the project to eleven provinces in the 1990s.[3] In the early 1990s, the Philippines radically devolved health services to district and local levels. Within India, several state-level experiments in decentralization have been carried out. Thus, a wide variety of combinations of the three decentralization forms can be seen around the world.

Another way of introducing health sector reforms is through introducing public-private partnership, contracting out and introducing new management structures so that the government's overburdened shoulders are relieved of the concerns of health needs of the people.

REFORMS IN KERALA

Over the years, decentralization and public-private partnership the approaches to health sector reforms have been partly or fully attempted in Kerala. As part of the democratic decentralization process in Kerala following the 73rd and 74th Constitutional Amendments, health sector was decentralized to a large extent. The process itself being a 'big bang', it had not considered in detail the scope, strategy to be adopted, and the changes expected specifically in health systems. The second approach is the donor-centred and -driven one where reforms are dependant on the kind of project support. In many such situations, these are also being tried out without 'diagnosing' the problems in the Kerala health system and without considering its strengths and weaknesses. As of now, we find a mixture of such approaches and initiatives running parallel to each other, making it difficult for each to reach a logical conclusion and impact.

THE KERALA HEALTH CRISIS

There are a number of disturbing trends in the situation of health in Kerala. Although Kerala's health indicators and access to health care are far better compared to most of the Third World populations, diseases such as malaria, once nearly eradicated, have begun staging comebacks. In addition to such communicable and infectious diseases which are staging comebacks, lifestyle diseases and degenerative diseases have begun to strain the health care system. These include cancer, heart disease, hypertension and other lifestyle disorders. In the meantime, the once acclaimed health care system has also failed to improve and get reoriented to address these challenges.

DECENTRALIZED PLANNING AND HEALTH SECTOR REFORMS IN KERALA

It was in this context that the decentralized planning process in Kerala, known as People's Campaign, for the Ninth Plan was initiated. How is it different from other experiences of decentralization in health sector? Why is it different?

The decentralization process in Kerala was not just part of the health sector reforms alone. It was part of the overall decentralization process following the 73rd and 74th Amendments to the Constitution of India. The planning process, which was unique to Kerala, also was not confined to health. In fact, the process covered almost all the development and service sectors where health was one among them. Many public health experts argue that health sector reforms cannot be considered in the realm of health sector alone as health by definition is the result of convergence of many a sector involving the major proximate determinants of health. For them, the decentralized planning process initiated in Kerala provides an ideal process where all the sectors, which contribute to health, are involved. On the other hand, it is argued that the reform had not focused on health sector nor it had any definite or specific strategies designed for health sector reforms.

Dennis Rondinelli, John R. Nellis and G. Shabbir Cheema, at the University of California, Berkeley Institute of International Studies had developed the conceptual framework of three types of decentralization: deconcentration, delegation, and devolution.[4] Deconcentration occurs when a central government ministry transfers some resources and/or decision-making power to a regional or local office. Delegation refers to the transfer of government authority over a particular set of tasks to other institutions such as state-owned enterprises. When the task is outsourced to a private sector enterprise it is called privatization, which in this schema is a form of delegation. The most substantial form of decentralization is devolution, in which authority is transferred to lower levels of government granting them some to all of the powers to plan, make decisions, raise revenues, employ staff, and monitor activities. This allows the lower levels to 'interact reciprocally with other units of government'. Kerala's decentralization experiment to some extent can be considered as devolution. There are differences too. Most of the powers mentioned have been transferred to the local bodies except for the powers to employ staff. Instead, the health care institutions along with the staff have been transferred to the local bodies. Thus, all the primary health centres have been transferred to the gram panchayats, community health centres to block panchayats, taluk hospitals to municipalities and district hospitals to district panchayats. Employees including the doctors of these institutions have also been transferred to the respective local bodies.

More than the powers to raise resources, the uniqueness of Kerala's decentralization process is the transfer of funds to the local bodies based on a comprehensive formula. In addition to the plan funds or the development funds, non-plan funds or the recurring and establishment cost funds are also transferred to the local bodies. Thus rather than shirking from the responsibilities in health sector, the state government has tried to empower the local self-governments by providing functions, functionaries and funds. Additional resource mobilization is not a mandatory responsibility as in the case where governments have withdrawn from the health sector, but provides scope for innovations in resource mobilization without affecting equity. Above all these, the process envisaged the people to be the decision makers, where the gram sabhas (village assemblies) have the powers to plan and monitor the various initiatives.

Gram sabhas listed the problems after which people's committees together with the elected representatives drew up projects that were prioritized by elected village and municipal council members. High levels of transparency have helped to reduce corruption and pilferage, thus leading to improvements in development sectors.

The experience with the decentralization process has been mixed in the health sector. We find that all the primary- and secondary-level health institutions and functionaries have been transferred to the local self-governments. One-third of the state's plan outlay (development funds) has also been made available to the local self-governments for preparing their own plans for various development and social sectors including health. This process by design is participatory with local people given the powers of decision-making. After eight years of implementation of the decentralization process, we find that the local self-governments were able to prepare plans, taking into consideration the needs and demands raised by the people. They were also able to address the proximate determinants of health like drinking water, sanitation, and housing. The process also brought to light various other mechanisms of additional resource mobilization without affecting equity which is the key word in Kerala's development. Access to and outreach of health services has definitely improved. There are various examples and models, though not universal across the state, of additional resource mobilization, public-private partnerships, strengthening of secondary-level institutions and disease prevention and comprehensive health delivery programmes under the leadership of local self-governments. Before going into the opinions of academicians and experts who have done a lot of studies on the process, this paper tries to enlist and analyse a few such experiences.

ADDITIONAL RESOURCE MOBILIZATION: THE NEDUMANGAD EXPERIENCE

Nedumangad Taluk Hospital serves a suburban area of the capital city of Thiruvananthapuram and its catchment area extends into the nearby hills where very low income and impoverished tribal households live. The taluk, or sub-district hospitals, are Kerala's second line of health care facilities after the local Primary Health Centres. Before 1996, the Nedumangad hospital had been in decline with a lack of adequate drinking water or latrine facilities, and outmoded and often non-functional medical equipment. The hospital's eight doctors attempted to treat 1,500 patients daily in a dilapidated outpatient room with a floor in need of major repairs. Catching the spirit of the campaign, local volunteers worked with the medical professionals to renovate the outpatient rooms, fix the drainage, sewage, and drinking water connections, improve the electrical wiring, and install new tables, chairs, beds, trolleys, sheets, and mattresses purchased with devolved funds. In connection with this work, the municipality set up a fair price store where medical products could be purchased at 10 per cent to 40 per cent below open market prices. As the hospital's basic infrastructure improved, it made more sense to invest in additional equipment. The municipality set up a blood bank and mortuary, renovated the maternity ward, and installed a new X-ray unit, ECG machine, and clinical laboratory. It also provided the funds to finish construction on a 100-bed expansion ward. The main improvements at Nedumangad were accomplished in four months. Free or very inexpensive medical services for some of the poorest households in the southern part of Kerala were upgraded to a much acceptable level of quality.

PUBLIC-PRIVATE PARTNERSHIP TO ADDRESS SECOND-GENERATION HEALTH PROBLEMS

While mentioning the crisis in health sector, the paper has already discussed some of the second-generation problems the state faces. The suicide rate of Kerala is three times higher than that of the national average. The rates of divorces and consumption of drugs are also increasing. In the case of severe mental diseases Kerala stands more or less equal to that of the national average. But, mental health care is the weakest part of public health care in Kerala.

Dr. Manoj Kumar Therayil who was a consultant psychiatrist at Edappal Hospitals (Pvt) Ltd. proposed a comprehensive community mental health care project for Ponnani block panchayat. He had done a number of studies about the mental health problems in Kerala earlier. In those studies he found that suicide rate in Ponnani region is much higher than other places. After a number of interactions and deliberations at different levels in the block panchayat, this project was included as a prime project in the health sector by the block panchayat in the 1998-9 plan. A 'Society for Community Mental Health' was formed by the block panchayat with the actors coming from both private and public health systems to coordinate different activities in this regard. 'Centre for Community Mental Health

Studies', a people's plan campaign initiative of Ponnani block panchayat, was started under the society.

It is interesting to note some of the activities under this initiative which have addressed those locally relevant issues which were not really addressed by the state public health system so far. These include 'adolescent marriage—an awareness programme'; school mental health programme addressing learning disabilities, suicide prevention activities, and mental health survey; addressing issues of old age health; and pain and palliative care initiatives. It is interesting to note how the public and private systems joined together in these initiatives, especially in the case of old age problems and pain and palliative care.

Old Age Problems: Some Solutions

In the mental health survey done by the health workers in the Ponnani block, it was found out that 25 per cent of old people need the help of others in one way or other. Five to ten per cent of old people are affected by dementia, which results in severe lack of memory. Our present-day society has not yet properly understood the needs and disabilities of old age people. Under the comprehensive community mental health care project, 'senior cards' that ensure life-long free consultation were distributed to the old people of Ponnani block. On producing the card free consultation will be available for them in all hospitals and in the houses of all doctors in this block area. The local unit of the Indian Medical Association (IMA) was also behind this project. A lot of old people among us have experience and knowledge in many fields. A number of 'old and young people meets' were held to help the elderly share their knowledge and experiences with young people and thereby making them feel useful to the society.

Severe lack of memory needs detailed consultation. Generally people don't consider this as a disease, regarding it as natural in old age. A 'Dementia Support Centre' was established in Ponnani block to give detailed treatment for memory problems, identification of dementia in the early stages and to give training to the family members to look after dementia patients. A small book, *Vardhakyam* (*Old Age*), which deals with healthy old age and dementia was published and made available to the people to make them aware of this subject.

Pain and Palliative Care Centre

'Santhwanam Pain and Palliative Care Society' was registered on 4 August 1999 as part of the people's plan programme and 'Santhwanam Pain and Palliative Care Centre' was started in Edappal. This is a joint venture of Ponnani block panchayat, Perumbadappu block panchayat, Ponnani municipality, four village panchayats of the Ponnani block and five village panchayats of Perumbadappu block with the help of the local branch of IMA. This centre was started in a building of Ponnani block panchayat.

STRENGTHENING SECONDARY-LEVEL INSTITUTIONS: THE MALAPPURAM DISTRICT HOSPITAL

Malappuram district hospital was established in 1942 as a government dispensary. It was developed into a taluk hospital (Eranad Taluk Hospital) in 1959. When Malappuram district was formed in 1969, the taluk hospital was converted to a district hospital. Actually the name board of the hospital was changed without any infrastructural development. A five-storeyed administrative block was inaugurated in 1990, but due to the rush of patients, four floors of this building were converted to general wards.

The poor people in the district had no other option but to seek medical facilities in the government hospitals. The facilities in PHCs, block PHCs, CHCs and taluk hospitals are not sufficient to meet the health care needs of common people. So a large number of people are coming to the district hospital directly without utilizing the local health care facilities. About 50 per cent of the cases coming to the district hospital are referral cases coming from other hospitals. But the district hospital is not equipped to meet the huge swell of patients in the most populous district in the state. The dilapidated buildings of the hospital shelter around 2,500 in-patients. More than 25,000 patients are treated monthly at the hospital. Malappuram has the largest population of women and children. In all other thirteen districts in Kerala there are district hospitals for women and children. But in Malappuram it has not materialized so far even though the state government in 1992 announced a project for a hospital for Rs. 1.68 crore.

As a part of the people's planning programme launched in Kerala in 1997 district hospitals were handed over to district panchayats on 1 July 1999. Malappuram district hospital was also handed over to the district panchayat the same day. The panchayat took the initiative and decided to confront the problem head on without resorting to the usual practice of pleading with the state government. The district panchayat convened a public meeting on 27 July 2001 at the district panchayat hall to discuss this matter. Three ministers and members of the legislative assembly from the district, district panchayat president and other members of district panchayat, heads of other local self-government institutions of the district, representatives of political parties and other organizations, the district collector and other district-level officials assembled to discuss this issue. The district panchayat decided to develop the hospital on its own by collecting funds from the people. The Malappuram District Hospital Welfare Council was formed for this purpose This 40-member council consists of all three ministers of the district, all elected representatives to the parliament and legislative assembly from the district, representatives of all political parties, representatives of local self-governments of the district and district-level officials.

The district panchayat prepared a two-stage developmental plan for the district hospital that cost Rs. 18 crore. The first stage of the developmental work will be completed in two years in an estimated cost of Rs. 8 crore. When the whole developmental work will be completed in five years it will be the first super specialty hospital in the government sector in the district. There will be 998 beds and all modern facilities for treating in-patients. Establishment of a mother and childcare centre operation theatre complex, trauma care unit, etc., will be major achievements of this development. The out-patient block will be constructed with all modern facilities. There will be a full-fledged laboratory, C.T. scan facility, X-ray unit and a modern blood bank. In the surgical block there will be twelve operation theatres, ICU, ICCU, modern maternity and childcare unit and post-delivery care centre. Special observation block for newborn babies, trauma care unit for treating accident cases and modern mortuary will be established. Uninterrupted water supply facilities and effective power supply system will be implemented. With the completion of the renovation work daily functioning of the hospital will be much more improved. There will be separate lifts for patients, staffs, and carrying hospital tools. There will be plants for processing bio-waste and wastewater. Facilities for parking vehicles will be available in the hospital compound. Large canteen, night shelter, nurses' quarters, etc., will also be constructed near the hospital.

The Malappuram district hospital welfare council constituted a welfare fund for the construction of a new hospital complex and made an appeal to all sections of people to donate liberally to this fund. The response from the public was tremendous. The society has turned the fund raising campaign for the hospital into a popular movement. All 14 blocks, 5 municipalities and 100 village panchayats of the district and district panchayat are donating their share in installments. All people's representatives including MPs, MLAs and representatives of all local self-governments in the district are donating their share also from the local development fund.

District panchayat had offered another Rs. 50 lakh from the next year's plan fund. Non-resident Indians offered Rs. 1 crore. So far Rs. 50 lakh has been collected from the public and Rs. 25 lakh from school children. This unparalleled initiative shown by the people of Malappuram resulted in the flow of contribution from all sections of people, organizations and institutions in the district. This helped in making the popular dream into a reality. Thus the district is on its way to becoming a role model for the state by masses joining hands in a historic mission.

INTERVENTION IN A PRIMARY HEALTH CENTRE: A DOCTOR FINDS AN OPPORTUNITY

Mangalapuram Primary Health Centre was inaugurated on 1 December 1978. For the next 20 years it was functioning as an ordinary PHC. There were only four rooms; people had to stand outside in hot sun and in rain for taking OP tickets. There was no waiting room for out-patients. Scarcity of clean water was a big problem as there was no pipe connection. The hospital staff were taking water from a deep well. One building that was constructed using the block fund was not being used. There was no compound wall for the hospital ground which is about one acre of land. It was being as a playground and as a grazing field for the cattle. There was no paved road but a mud track connecting the main road to the hospital.

Dr. Najeeb, a young and energetic doctor, joined the Mangalapuram PHC in 1995. From the beginning itself he was of the opinion that this PHC needed to be developed since it was situated near the National Highway. But he was reluctant to take any initiative on account of his bitter experience regarding the construction of a compound wall in the PHC where he had worked earlier.

During this time the People's Plan Programme was launched in the state. In the beginning Dr. Najeeb viewed it with a lot of doubt, which were subsequently cleared through training programmes. He began dreaming of developing the PHC with the developmental mechanism of uniting the people and ensuring their participation. He decided to change his attitude and join the people's movement. He actively participated in gram sabhas and developmental seminars.

In both forums, people raised a lot of issues related to the health sector, which had needed to be solved. The doctor proposed a multi-point programme that included steps for providing basic medical needs, understanding problems of the people and implementing new health programmes, preparing oneself for these activities and creating a positive outlook in the employees of the PHC, and organizing a voluntary group to work in the society. Financial constraints prevented solving all the problems together. But the People's Plan Programme opened the door for that. The power given to the local self-governments for additional resource mobilization from different sources was a big opportunity. It was also a challenge.

Money from the plan fund, MP, fund, panchayat fund, help from the health and science and technology departments, voluntary work, donation by people, help from the Rotary Club,

Lion's Club, merchant and trader organizations, cooperatives, local clubs, services of expert doctors from medical colleges, various departments, professional groups from abroad were channelized for the development of PHC in this small village. The PHC was developed into a centre with computer and Internet facilities and a mental rehabilitation centre with cable TV and other amenities.

The acceptance and active participation of people and the panchayat opened the way for new activities. The Centre for Disease Prevention and Awareness (CDPA), Need-Oriented Health Action (NOHA), horticultural projects in the premises of the Hospital, and labour rehabilitation project are some of these activities.

GRAM PANCHAYAT OPENS A HOSPITAL

In a suburb of Ernakulam campaign activists organized a strong movement for the construction of a cooperative hospital. The process of planning and building the hospital involved participation by more than one hundred neighbourhood groups that sent proposals to the gram sabhas that met twice yearly as part of the campaign. The panchayat committee put up Rs. 50,000 as a startup subsidy that was followed by 1,221 residents who purchased memberships at Rs. 250 each. Seeing such substantial community support, the panchayat committee offered a section of the compound next to the cultural centre and library. Construction began in 1998. On 13 June 1999 the hospital opened with a daytime out-patient service, two GPs, an internist, and a paediatrician. Three nurses, one lab technician, and a pharmacist constituted the medical support staff. Within the first week of operation, member-patients and their families began demanding that the physicians offer night hours. The hospital staff rearranged their schedules to meet the felt needs. Two additional doctors were hired, and five beds were made available for patients needing hospital care.

Six months later, there were fourteen beds, a dermatologist, and an ENT doctor who came in two days a week. A female gynaecologist in the area volunteered her services for certain emergencies. In the third year of the people's campaign, the panchayat committee purchased an X-ray machine. In June 1999 the hospital had been receiving 100 visits per day; by October 2001 the number had risen to 250. Membership in the hospital cooperative society had grown to 2,600. There were 21 doctors on staff, 8 of them full-time. In 2002 plans were made to expand the 60-bed hospital to 200 beds by 2008. In November 2001 the hospital reached the break—even point in fee *versus* expenses. It is not intended to make a profit, but there are hopes for raising additional donations from the public to expand some services.

A nine-member committee democratically elected by the votes of the hospital members who have purchased at least one share manages the Thrikkakkara Cooperative Hospital. No matter how many shares one owns, it is one shareholder one vote. In 2002 the directors included one physician, a former district medical officer, a local businessman, a lawyer, a social worker, an elected official of the block panchayat, two political activists, and one former panchayat committee member. Hospital fees are intentionally kept about 40 per cent below private sector charges, and cooperative members receive an additional 10 per cent reduction. Physicians recruited to the staff are asked to accept below-market salaries for full-time work or to do at least some part-time work at the hospital.

In addition to its in-house medical functions, Thrikkakkara Cooperative Hospital conducts substantial outreach programmes to improve the public health in the surrounding area. Projects include mobile check-up teams to poor neighbourhoods, seminars on drinking water and waste control, classes on ORT, and work with local environmental groups. The hospital has installed a solar generator and a rainwater-holding tank, and is recycling its non-medical waste through a vermi (worm) process developed in Kerala to speed up the transformation of sewage and garbage into fertilizer that can be sold to local farmers.

COMPREHENSIVE HEALTH IMPROVEMENT PROGRAMME

Near the central Kerala town of Kottayam, the citizens of Erattupettah village became especially active in a comprehensive health project that suggests a model for the future for other

Kerala communities. Based on their awareness of numerous sanitation problems in the village, residents formed a 21-person 'healthy village committee'. In 1998, they carried out a basic health survey of the village, finding that 827 houses (20 per cent) lacked proper latrines, only 16 per cent of houses had private wells, the PHC was in need of major repairs, and many restaurants and tea shops were dumping waste and sewage directly into the two rivers passing through the village. Of sixteen water samples taken, only two were free of E. coli that causes stomach problems, 15 per cent of babies were born with birth weight below 2,500 gm, and many children remained without basic vaccinations despite high state average.

To correct these problems, campaign activists mobilized public opinion and action resulting in Rs. 2.4 million in local resources that added 36 per cent to the Rs. 4.2 million brought in to the comprehensive health project from the devolved funds. The PHC received major repairs. A school health programme resulted in 6,000 students in the nine local schools getting checkups and health identity cards. The local taluk hospital doctors and the PHC staff then expanded the school health cards project to include all residents. The 44 teashops and restaurants were visited and citations issued; 36 of them fixed the sewage and waste removal problems and got new health licenses. Restaurant employees were checked for diseases and given health certificates. The attention to public eating and drinking places seems especially important in view of a 1998-9 study in southern Kerala that showed significantly increased chances of contracting diarrhoea after eating out as opposed to cooking or making tea at home. Over a four-year period, 658 sanitary latrines were constructed, 80 per cent of the number needed. Safe water was brought to 1,750 houses, 88 per cent of those in need. In addition to private homes, bus stations and markets got new latrines and bathing facilities, an important improvement in a village that has many transient workers in trade and travellers passing through to nearby pilgrimage sites. A village garbage collection site was established in an area far from houses. Although no statistical follow-up was done, local health workers reported in interviews that the disease rate seems to have come down compared to adjacent villages.

THE RESULTS AND IMPACT

All over the world, it has been difficult to measure the potential of decentralization. But certain evidences show that over the initial five years of the campaign, PHCs were improved in hundreds of localities. Physicians and community activists worked together, improving relations among them as exemplified in the Thrikkakkara Cooperative Hospital or Mangalapuram PHC or other examples cited earlier. One of the most important areas was the taluk hospitals where block panchayats and municipalities put in equipment and local committees provided voluntary labour. Along with the Nedumangad case described earlier, taluk hospitals in Changanassery, Vaikom, and Aluva underwent major upgrades and most others experienced some improvements. The lowest income sections of the population were encouraged to make more use of the less expensive public sector facilities. Usage of PHCs and taluk hospitals also increased.

Overall, the decentralization process with emphasis on decentralized planning helped to institute a more direct accountability of public health and health care institutions, with the local bodies taking up the responsibility in managing health care institutions as is evident from the examples given above. Though these examples give some insight into additional resource mobilization, it is yet to be studied whether the resources were managed more efficiently. There definitely are better linkages between information and planning, especially information regarding local issues and potentials being used for health sector planning. Though the examples cited above show some indications regarding the ability to respond effectively to the variety of different needs and capacities of different regions and localities, it is yet to be proven that there is easier inter-agency coordination.

D. Narayana and Hari Kurup in their study 'Decentralization of Health Care Sector in Kerala: Some Issues' have pointed out that the elected representatives are conversant with reform issues in health, like role of non-government health care services, charging user fee, management of hospitals, levels of service, and so on.[5] V. Ramankutty in the paper 'Health Planning and Decentralization: The Kerala Experience' says that the local governments have an increased space and enhanced range of choices in respect of planning in general and health in particular. However these are not realized due to limitations like lack of expertise, and absence of full involvement by doctors.[6] Study by Varadarajan et al., shows that resource allocation is not adequate for the health sector and even the limited resource is divided among smaller health projects. But there is evidence of high marginal effects.[7]

WEAKNESSES

Though a few successful models have been presented, these are not be considered as universal phenomena. In fact, though the decentralization process provided scope for such interventions, such interventions have not happened across the state on a large scale. Moreover, the issue of sustainability of such interventions is also being questioned now. Beyond its own internal weaknesses, Kerala's radical decentralization suffered from its inability to decentralize the bureaucracy in the way it should have. Various disease prevention activities are run through the Central Government programmes without considering the local realities. PHC and taluk hospital physicians and other staff are paid by the state and not by the local communities. Transfer of staff is thus beyond the scope of the local governments. In their efforts to provide better medical care, the local governments could add a new examination room to a PHC but they could not, due to obvious reasons, directly intervene to improve the quality of actual delivery of clinical services. They also had problems assuring the supply of medicines. Some communities took charge of this by assisting the PHCs in collecting needed items from government supply depots.

On the other hand, decentralization could not bring in much visible improvement in the quality of services rendered through public health system. Local self-governments have not been able to professionally manage the health institutions transferred to them. This is related to the lack of functional role differentiation, skills and lack of a management system. This is evident from the issue of dual control where the state department has the technical control and the local self-governments have the administrative control. Transfers and postings are with the department. Purchase of drugs and equipment are still centralized. This leads to the question of 'loyalty'—to the department or to the local self-government, which invariably has affected the smooth and efficient running of the health institutions. Health is a technical subject where there is need for expertise to plan at the local level and where public preference alone would not suffice.

Some of the shortfalls are due to poor planning for decentralization, inefficiency of community-based monitoring system, conflicts between centralized health department and local bodies, problems of staff assignment and salaries, failure to allocate adequate resources to the decentralized units, lack of public engagement, vagueness about the meaning of decentralization, and a variety of other factors. Another key aspect of decentralization is the unit or level to which the decentralization goes. To fulfil the promise of decentralization, should one decentralize to the district, the sub-district, the municipality, the village, or the neighbourhood? Which kinds of health services and institutions should be controlled at which levels? Should some remain centralized? These questions remain unanswered in part because of the lack of systematic data, and in part because the answers may vary from society to society owing to variations in local demographic, economic, cultural, and political circumstances and to the types of health problems most in need of attention.

OTHER REFORM INITIATIVES

Parallel to this, there are attempts at centralized health sector reforms. This is mainly based on the state's initiatives to bring in donors and resources so as to tackle the fiscal crisis through which it has been passing through over the last several years. Noteworthy among these are the proposed and evolving programmes in secondary and tertiary health system development projects. While there are well-documented studies on idle capacities and idle infrastructure and facilities in the health institutions in the state, the new initiatives have ignored this so much so that the thrust is again on infrastructure and facilities. There is also mention of new initiatives in resource mobilization including user fee and insurance. But, the details are yet to be worked out. Another major initiative is in the form of Service Delivery Improvement Project (SDIP) under the Modernizing Government Programme (MGP) with assistance from Asian Development Bank. This tries to bring together the local self-governments and the state health department to improve service delivery in a few selected institutions.

Over the years, Kerala has also developed models in community participation through Hospital Development Committees (HDC), which are similar to Rogi Kalyan Samitis. Though functioning of these HDCs have not been studied in detail, there are anecdotal evidences to show that they have been able to prevent to some extent the total decline of the public health system. HDC consists of representatives of the community, hospital, state and the concerned local self-government. These have been able to mobilize resources through systems similar to user fee. Resources mobilized thus are being used for improving the facilities in hospitals. The effectiveness and efficiency of these committees vary from place to place and from institution to institution. HDCs, being not part of the health system *per se*, have not been able to contribute much to the improvement in quality of services nor to the improvement in management of these hospitals.

CONCLUSION

There are issues of concern that need to be addressed. Many of the initiatives discussed were not introduced as health sector reforms to address the crisis in the Kerala health system. There was never a motivation nor the political will for the state to introduce comprehensive health sector reforms for addressing these issues. Some of the reforms are being introduced for the sake of reforms, catering to the needs of the donors rather than the people. There has been no scientific analysis of the health system, where the strengths and weaknesses of the already widely distributed public health system in Kerala have been overlooked. While Kerala boasts of its achievements in health, and also of its well-distributed accessible public health system, what the state faces is more complex than what it is in other Indian states. Deteriorating quality of services, more than three-fourths of the health budget being spent on meeting recurring expenses on salaries and establishment, and the overall fiscal crisis of the state are concerns for Kerala too. In addition, Kerala has to address the second-generation problems in health sector. These have roots in epidemiological and demographic transition, health awareness of the population, the impact of growing private sector and growing influence of medical technology. This calls for health sector reforms. Decentralization in the health system needs to be strengthened, but not in isolation. It has to be integrated with the multilevel planning process. The centralized state system needs to focus more on improving the tertiary health care sector. Various means of additional resource mobilization needs to be explored taking lessons from some of the experiences of the decentralization process and HDCs. The effort should also be in ensuring equity in which Kerala has its strength. Private-public partnerships are to be developed to address these concerns in the pattern a few local self-governments has developed. In fact, these reforms need not pave the way for the government to withdraw from health sector. It could be for a more active involvement of the governments, including the local self-governments, in providing better, effective and efficient accessible health care to the people. This also needs proper integration of the various interventions in health sector that calls for a comprehensive health policy.

NOTES

* This paper has freely adopted many of the observations mentioned in the paper 'Decentralization of Health Services: The Kerala People's Campaign', prepared by the author along with Richard W. Franke and B. Ekbal. It along with all the case studies included in the present paper were prepared as part of the research conducted by the three on 'Local Planning and Democratic Participation as Mechanisms for Improving Third World Health Conditions: Recent Experiments in Kerala, India', with grant from the John D. and Catherine T. MacArthur Foundation. We received valuable research assistance from Suresh Kumar S. and from Mariamma Sanu George. We also express our thanks to the elected representatives and the volunteers of the People's Campaign who not only generated the data for this study but gave generously of their time to assist us in our research.

The paper has also adopted many views expressed in the note 'Decentralization and Reproductive Health' by S.M. Vijayanand.

1. Iain W. Aitken, 'Implementation and Integration of Reproductive Health Services in a Decentralized System', in Kolehmainen-Aitken, and Riitta-Liisa, eds., *Myths and Realities about the Decentralization of Health Systems*, Boston: Management Sciences for Health, 1999.
2. Charles C. Stover, 'Financing, Service Delivery, and Decentralization in the Philippines and Kenya', in Kolehmainen-Aitken and Riitta-Liisa, eds., *Myths and Realities about the Decentralization of Health Systems*, Boston: Management Sciences for Health, 1999.
3. Thomas Bossert, R. Soebekti and Nyoman Kumara Rai, 'Bottom-up Planning in Indonesia: Decentralization in the Ministry of Health', *Health Policy and Planning*, 1991.
4. Dennis A. Rondinelli, John R. Nellis and G. Shabbir Cheema, 'Decentralization in Developing Countries: A Review of Recent Experience', World Bank Staff Working Papers Number 581, Washington D.C., 1984.
5. D. Narayana and Hari Kurup, 'Decentralization of Health Care Sector in Kerala: Some Issues', Kerala: Centre for Development Studies, 2000.
6. V. Ramankutty, 'Health Planning and Decentralization: The Kerala Experience', unpublished report.
7. D. Varadarajan, K.R. Thankappan and Jayapalan Sabeena, 'Strengthening PHCs through Panchayati Raj: A Situational Analysis of PHCs in Kerala', Kerala: Achutha Menon Centre for Health Sciences Studies, 2001.

CHAPTER 4

Access to Medicines in Public Health Care: Lessons from Tamil Nadu

N. LALITHA

1. THE CONCEPT OF ESSENTIAL DRUGS[1]

According to the recent report on access to medicines, one-third of the world's population does not have access to basic and essential drugs and this figure rises to one half if the poorest parts of Africa and Asia are considered (Dukes and Paula, 2004). Though the disease patterns may vary in and developing countries, one common problem that prevails in such countries is the inadequate access to medicines. Keeping in mind that medicines are important in curing and preventing diseases, the ultimate goal of 'Health for All' cannot be achieved if people do not have adequate access to essential drugs. It is an ironical fact that a high proportion of deaths/ailments in the developing world is preventable/curable in principle with the available medicines, though accessibility is restricted due to factors such as cost of the drug, purchasing power of the people, physical availability of the medicine in the market and health care centres, and so on. Where government is involved in providing the medicines, accessibility can be impeded by lack of funding, inappropriate procurement and selection, and lack of prioritization due to absence of data regarding the demand for the right medicines. In the absence of this crucial data, government's meagre resources are spent on unnecessary piling of drugs, which might not be used within their shelf life at all.

Accessibility to medicines is increasingly debated in the context of: (a) structural adjustment programmes introduced by various government that resulted in reduction in social expenditures; (b) growing globalization of trade; (c) exclusive rights provided to the inventors of medicines and (d) the growing inequity in health between the North and South. These issues have made the governments to concentrate more on providing access to medicines to the needy. While access to patented medicines is a complex issue, access to off-patented essential drugs has been initiated through spearheading the concept of essential drugs by the WHO and drug donations through bilateral agreements.

The concept of essential drugs refers to those drugs that satisfy the health care needs of a majority of the population and therefore need to be made available in adequate quantity and at a price that individuals and the community can afford. WHO, created in 1946, earlier limited its role in the field of medicines to the standards of manufacturing and quality control. Later it went on to advocating drugs that are safe and affordable and that would meet the health requirements of the Third World and thus, the concept of essential drugs was introduced. The first list of essential drugs consisted of 224 drugs and many countries drew their list of formulary from this template. The WHO list is frequently modified reviewing the health scenario of different countries.

At the beginning of the year 2000 as many as 198 countries had adopted the WHO's list of essential drugs. Medicines, which account for 10 to 30 per cent of public spending for health in most countries, are the most promising area for efficiency gains. Very large savings can be achieved by improving the selection and quantification of drug requirements in part through the use of essential national drug lists and by purchasing drugs competitively. Evidence documented by WHO shows that as a result of adopting a rational drug approach, countries have cut down the drug costs within the health expenditure and because of improved availability of drugs in public utilities public utilization and image of the utilities have improved.

As far as India is concerned, though there exists a national drug list, different states have their own list of formulary that is not necessarily based on the national list of essential drugs. Tamil Nadu, Delhi, Maharashtra, Andhra Pradesh, Himachal Pradesh, Karnataka, Punjab, Rajasthan, Uttar Pradesh, Madhya Pradesh, Orissa and West Bengal are some of the states that have taken initiatives towards adopting a rational drug approach. Figure 4.1 shows the status of the WHO-India Essential Drugs Programme in 2002. As evident, not all the states have adopted a wholistic approach or an approach as propaganded by WHO. Hence, there could be differences in their achievements in terms of operationalizing the essential drug list across different health care in a state, rationalizing their budget expenditure, and making medicines available in public health utilities. In this paper, we focus on the efforts of the Tamil Nadu (herein referred to as TN) government in adopting a rational drugs approach to provide supplies to its government-supported health care system. Before we actually discuss this process a brief note on social spending of TN will be apt for understanding the reform measures, which is presented in Section 2 of this paper. Section 3 presents the pre-reform scenario regarding medicinal supply in TN. Section

FIGURE 4.1: PROGRESS IN THE WHO-INDIA ESSENTIAL DRUGS PROGRAMME 1997-2001

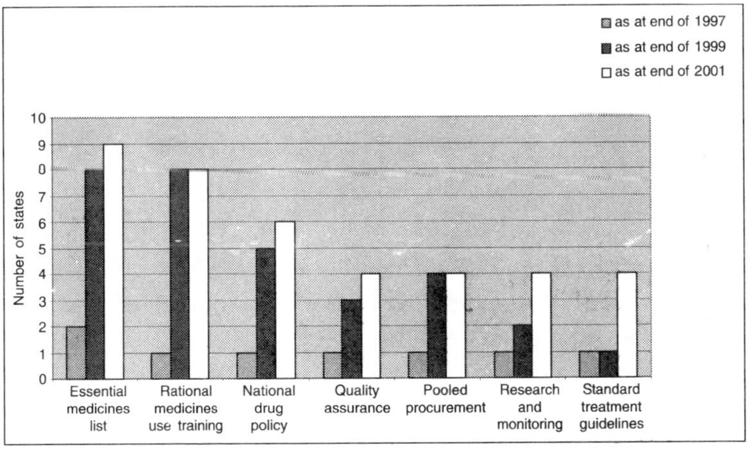

Source: Annual Report 2001, *Essential Drugs and Medicines Policy: Extending the Evidence Base*, World Health Organization.

4 and its various subsections discuss the details of the government efforts in supplying rational drugs to its various health care systems. Section 5 discusses impact of adopting a rational drug approach. The replicability of TNMSC model is presented in section 6. This section is followed by the conclusion.

2. SOCIAL SPENDING IN TAMIL NADU

Social spending by states, i.e. allocation on education, health, water supply and sanitation, depends on the social priorities of the state and there are obvious differences observed in the social spending of the states. However, expenditure on medical and public health expenditure for any state ranks next to the expenditure on education (Lalitha, 1998). This expenditure however includes salaries, administration, capital expenditure and medicines. Because of such continued allocation, a huge infrastructure of government health care is available in India to provide health facilities, which range from hospitals for specialized treatments and research to preventive health care in rural areas. However as Dreze and Sen (1995) observe

> India has poor health achievements despite spending a comparatively large part of its GNP on health (if the public and private spending is added). Much of the mismatch between the resources and achievements is due to the functioning of the public health care system especially in rural areas. In some states, this system is little more than a collection of deserted primary health centres, filthy dispensaries, unmotivated doctors and chaotic hospitals. (p. 101)

Traditionally, while states with higher growth and higher per capita income spend more on social services such as education, health, nutrition and water supply as compared to the states with less income and are still developing, yet some of the states are able to target their social spending to get the desired effects. A few authors have observed that social spending in southern states is better targeted than other states. Particularly the experience of southern states such as Kerala, Tamil Nadu and Andhra Pradesh in targeting health subsidies (Mahal et al., 2003) and public distribution system respectively has been the focus of many studies. Dreze and Sen (1995) point out that 'most of the initiatives in social security measures taken in south Indian states were in the context of electoral politics'. They point out that by contrast in large north Indian states social security and related issues have little place in party programmes and electoral debates. And little time is wasted on real issues such as undernutrition, illiteracy, unemployment or ill health. Particularly, TN's emphasis on human development rather than human resource development and its positive impact on poor clearly emerge in the works of Guhan (1989) and Seeta Prabhu (2001).

Despite the high unemployment and the prevalence of casual labour, the government did not take recourse to schemes such as employment guarantee scheme. It appears that since transfers via wage payments *per se* are an expensive and inefficient approach to helping poor (hence) welfare programmes for SC and ST, basic needs provision and social assistance are likely to be more cost effective (Guhan, 1995). Tamil Nadu follows this by allocating more to social protectionist measures rather than to employment creation programmes. For instance, the midday meal scheme started as a voluntary scheme with contributions from local people but was soon adopted by the government. Over the years it has covered other targeted groups of people like children between 2-15 years, pregnant women and pensioners. Besides directly benefiting the targeted population, the labour-intensive nature of the programme opened up several employment opportunities for destitute women. Similarly, old-age pensions were introduced in 1962, two years after the formation of TN as a separate state. It still continues and the coverage has been extended to cover widows and handloom weavers.

An important distinction between the schemes announced by TN and the central government schemes such as IRDP is that, in the latter because of the ceiling on the overall budget, if the non-poor get a larger share, then the eligible poor do not get the benefits. But in TN schemes all those who are eligible benefit by such schemes and hence a non-poor getting a benefit doesn't exclude an eligible poor getting the benefits (Guhan, 1988). Though such expenditures have their budget implications, successive governments have added or continued such schemes, mainly for maintaining their 'pro poor' image and because of the positive impact of such schemes, on primary education and health. Due to large government efforts through various health campaigns, people of TN have become vocal regarding their basic rights and do not shy away in bringing any lapses to the notice of the authorities who are thereby forced to take action. The decision to revamp the system of procurement of medicines for the government health care system was also as a result of public outcry about the non-availability and shortage of medicines in the government health care sector, which is detailed below.

3. THE PRE-REFORM SCENARIO

Until 1995, the responsibility to procure and supply drugs to the TN government health care was with the 'Centralized Purchasing Committee' (CPC). Some of the state governments follow this type of procurement even now. In TN, the CPC functioned under the chairmanship of the health secretary and comprised the three heads of directorate's, viz., Directorate of Medical Service, Directorate of Medical Education and Directorate of Public Health. The CPC used to invite tenders. The requirement in the tender was based on the demand for drugs arrived at by consolidating the requirements of all the institutions that are meant for providing medical care in the state (Figure 4.2). For PHCs and taluka hospitals, the drug indents were consolidated and orders were placed at the district level. In the invitation to tender, preference was first given to public sector units, and if they failed to meet the demand, then private manufacturers were approached, which obviously meant delay in the supply of medicines. Hence, when the system was changed to that of inviting tenders for the supply of medicines, competitive prices were achieved but supply continued to suffer because tenders were given without regard to the units' production capacity and quality of the products. Rent-seeking behaviour was not uncommon. Understandably in this situation, supplies did not arrive on time. All this resulted in acute shortage of medicines in the government health services. Hence, to meet the demand, drugs were bought from the open market at higher prices and hospitals themselves placed orders directly with the suppliers, which meant different prices prevailed for the same drug.

FIGURE 4.2: HEALTH SECTOR OF TAMIL NADU

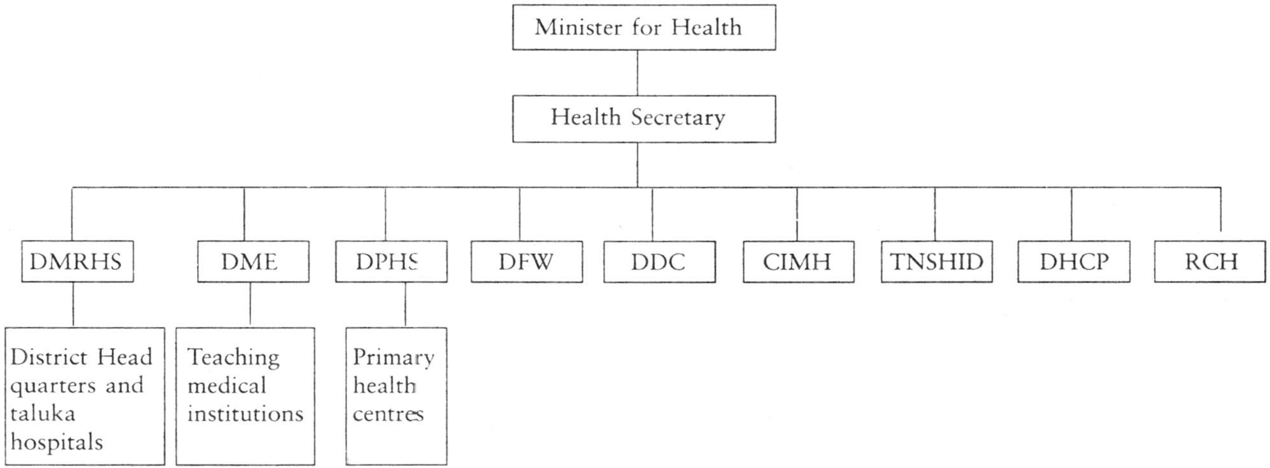

DMRHS	Directorate of Medical and Rural Health Services
DME	Directorate of Medical Education
DPH	Directorate of Public Health and Preventive Medicines
DFW	Directorate of Family Welfare
DDC	Directorate of Drugs Control
CIMH	Commissionerate of Indian medicine and Homeopathy
TNSHTD	Tamil Nadu State Health Transport Department
DHCP	DANIDA Health Camp Project
RCH	Reproductive and Child Health Project

A major shortfall of this system was that it resulted in buying and stocking a lot of irrational and unnecessary drugs of poor quality, because the procurement was based on consolidation of requirements of all the hospitals and was not with reference to any list. About 1,000 drugs were in use and no scrutiny was made about the therapeutical use of each drug that was bought. Further, medicines were bought in their brand names in bulk but in loose packing. Even dealers and stockists could apply for tender and supply to the hospitals. Showing favours to a particular company was not uncommon and no scrutiny was made about the firms selected to supply the drugs. This resulted in very small firms getting huge bulk orders and who were not in a position to supply on a timely basis. In this chaotic situation, hospitals reeled in shortage of drugs and patients had the option of either buying the medicines from the open market, which they were supposed to get free of cost, or going without medicines. Poornalingam (1998) aptly describes this situation:

> The concept of budgetary control was unknown to the hospitals. They (the concerned authorities) indented for drugs without any reference to the budget allocation. As a result, the overall budget allocation for the department was exhausted quite early, and non-availability of funds was then cited as the reason for the shortage of drugs, whereas drugs not immediately required were stocked in large quantities. No one had any idea of the stock position. A particular drug would be in short supply in a hospital despite a surplus stock in another hospital. The district and state level officials in charge of drug procurement and distribution did not have any information about the stock position of any drug. If they wanted any such information, they had to collect it from all the institutions. By the time the information was received, it would become outdated. Pilferage and wastage of drugs were common. Since there was overstocking of drugs in some hospitals and a regular mechanism to transfer such excess stocks to needy places was not routinely available (and hence) some drugs became time-barred and were wasted. (pp. 101-2)

While this method resulted in exhausting the budget allocated for medicines, essential drugs and drugs that are used for common ailments and surgical items were highly inadequate, which resulted in public outcry. Several of the print media carried news stories on the rent-seeking behaviour in the purchase of drugs and highlighted the shortfall of drugs in government health care system. This resulted in government taking some stern action. As a result of this, the old system was completely dismantled. A new administration started working on improved ways of procuring and distributing drugs. This paved way for the setting up of the Tamil Nadu Medical Services Corporation.

4. THE REFORM MEASURES

The WHO recommends that any governmental effort to provide access to medicines has to take care of the following four crucial factors (1) sustainable finance; (2) affordable prices; (3) rational selection of drugs and use and (4) reliable system of medicine supply (quoted in Dukes and Paula, 2004). In other words, when the government is involved in the supply of drugs, it has to ensure that it does not suffer from (a) inadequate buying practices; (b) improper estimation of demand for drug; (c) inefficient procurement and distribution of drugs; (d) and irrational prescription. All these flaws lead to improper utilization of the budget allocation with the net result being less value received for the amount spent by the government/consumer. Hence, different countries have adopted different methods to supply drugs.[2] These are: (1) central medical stores, (2) autonomous supply agency, (3) direct delivery system, (4) primary distributor system and (5) fully private supply. In India models of central medical stores and autonomous supply agencies are prevalent among a few states. The Central Medical Stores (CMS) approach is followed by some of the states in India and countries like Ghana, Oman and Zimbabwe. In this, drugs are financed, procured and distributed by the government which is the owner, funder and manager of the entire system. Selection, procurement and distribution are all handled by a unit within the health ministry. This is a logical approach if the medicines are all imported through one channel. However, CMS's have experienced problems with financial management, quantification of requirements, management of tenders, warehouse management, and transport and security of drugs. These problems have been exacerbated by political or administrative influences and weak financial discipline.

Autonomous supply agencies are constituted as parastatals, either under the ministry of health or as independent organizations with boards of directors including representation from other (than health) government ministries. Their primary and priority client is government health services and they may or may not operate on a non-profit basis. Examples of countries that have adopted this are Benin, Haiti, Sudan, Tanzania, Uganda and Zambia. The board is autonomous in running the agency but reports to a higher official from the ministry of health who may be involved in the appointment of the chairman of the board or the executive officer. The purpose of establishing an autonomous supply agency is to achieve the efficiency and flexibility associated with private management and private sector employment conditions. At the same time, presence of the public sector is also maintained to ensure that the autonomous services provide a range of essential drugs at reasonable prices with adequate control of quality. The basic concept is that under the right conditions, a well-constituted management board or board of directors will have the freedom to appoint qualified senior managers who will in turn ensure an efficient and accountable supply agency. Features that will ensure success of autonomous service models are: (1) supervision by an independent management board; (2) professional pharmaceutical supply managers; (3) adequate financing; (4) public accountability and sound financial management; (5) focus on essential drugs; (6) focus on quality assurance, both in terms of products and of services provided.

While many of these features of an autonomous supply agency have been incorporated in giving shape to the Tamil Nadu Medical Services Corporation (TNMSC) set up by the TN government to manage the entire drug delivery system, yet it is difficult to pinpoint whether it is based on any particular model.[3] The credit goes to the team of bureaucrats and technocrats who had the vision to meticulously plan and implement the activities and a supportive government, which was willing to introduce the reform measures.

Organizational Set Up of TNMSC

TNMSC was set up as an autonomous corporation in July 1994 under the Companies Act of 1956, for the purpose of supplying essential drugs and services. It commenced its services to buy, store and distribute drugs and medicines in January 1995. The health secretary of the Tamil Nadu government is the chairman of TNMSC. An officer from the Indian Administrative Service is posted as the managing director and looks after the day-to-day operations of TNMSC. Compared to any government office, which usually has huge manpower, TNMSC works with skeleton staff (Figure 4.3). There is hardly any permanent employee of TNMSC, except for the company secretary, who functions as chief accounts officer; all others are on deputation from other government departments. The staff in-charge of Electronic Data Processing (EDP) are employees of the company that has established the computer network. This arrangement helps in keeping the overheads and administrative expenditures to a minimum. Currently TNMSC supplies drugs to the following institutions: government teaching medical colleges and hospitals; district headquarters and taluka headquarters hospitals; all primary health centres and through them the health sub-centres; juvenile homes; ESI hospitals; all prisons and police department hospitals; cooperative sugar factories and tea plantations; government dispensaries; veterinary hospitals, road transport corporation hospitals; and all local body hospitals.

Selection of Drugs and Quantification

The root cause of problems in government supplies is that often there is lack of identification of appropriate drugs and lack of quantification, which has been detailed in an earlier section. Hence, the first task in the hands of TNMSC was to identify medicinal needs and arrive at a list of essential drugs. For this purpose, a drug committee consisting of professors of medicine, pharmacology, therapeutics, a representative from WHO, health secretary and the managing director of TNMSC was formed. After detailed discussions and looking at the prevailing morbidity pattern and the diseases calendar prevailing in different areas of the state, a list of 240 generic drugs was arrived at. A VED—Vital, Essential, Desired—analysis of drugs was also carried out in the selection of the drugs. Vital are the important drugs needed for a disease; essential are those identified by the WHO for the disease; and desired drugs are those suggested by the deans and heads of the departments to be included in the list.

FIGURE 4.3: ORGANIZATIONAL STRUCTURE OF TNMSC

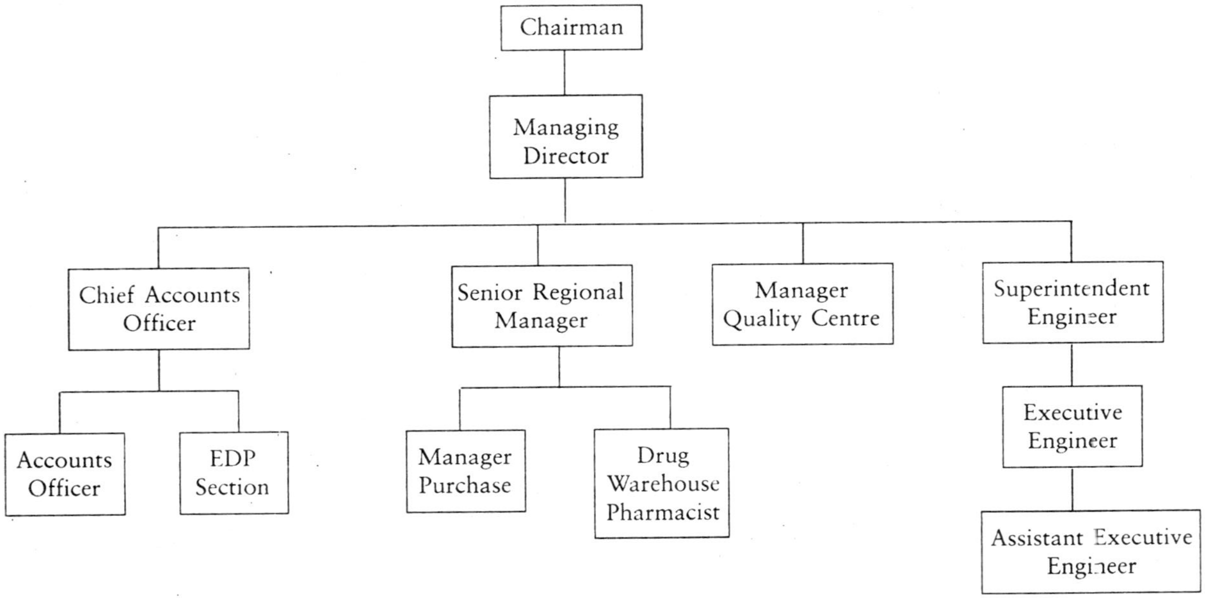

Source: TNMSC

Sticking to the WHO recommendation that the drugs should be of single drug ingredient and not multiple combinations except a few, TNMSC does not have combination drugs. The problem with multiple combinations is that they have side-effects and it is difficult to identify the cause of such side-effects. Quantifying the demand for drugs proved to be difficult for the task committee because, under the previous system hospitals were buying drugs without any accurate assessment. So in the initial days, the drug committee procured drugs on a rough estimate and over a period of time it was stabilized. However, now from the movement of drugs from the warehouse, the demand for a drug is arrived at and drugs are transferred from one place to another if there is more demand in a particular place. Besides this, computerization has also made it possible to monitor any particular health units' over- or under-use of allocation of drugs.

Besides selecting the drugs, the drug committee also worked out the cost of each medicine, taking into consideration the costs of raw material and manufacturing cost, cost of packing, excise duty paid, and a certain minimum profit margin. This exercise was also useful in identifying the quality of the drugs. For instance, if the raw materials have been bought from places of dubious quality then the supplier can quote very less price. However, if the supplies have been brought from qualified suppliers then the prices cannot go beyond a certain level.

Another important decision that was taken by the committee was to do away with the earlier practice of procuring and dispensing the drugs in loose, which reduces the quality of the medicine and its impact on the disease. The committee decided to get the supplies in aluminium foils and blister packs, syrups in 60 ml or 40 ml packs and ointments in small 5-gm or 10 gm tubes. This also helped in avoiding wastages and preventing the reduction in the shelf life of the drug in store. Most importantly, it helped in improving the image of the public health care system among people, since they were getting medicines, which 'looked the same as the ones that were brought from the pharmacy'. Incidentally, according to a survey done in TN in the year 2000, 20 per cent of the 50 best-selling drugs in the private drug outlets were also on the drug list of TNMSC. In order to avoid pilferages, it was also stipulated that all the tablets and capsules carry the logo TG meaning 'Tamil Nadu Government' and the message that the said drug is meant for the supplies of Tamil Nadu government and not meant for sale. Sutures do not bear the logo since it is difficult to emboss the logo on them.

FINANCIAL RESOURCE ALLOCATION

Reallocation of financial resources meant for the purchase of drugs from the institutions to TNMSC is one of the reform measures and hence TNMSC does not have a separate budget allocation to carry out its activities. Table 4.1 provides the allocation towards health expenditure by the TN government and expenditure on drugs by the three directorates, viz.,

TABLE 4.1: BUDGET FOR HEALTH 2002-4

(*Rs. in crores*)

Particulars	*2002-3 (RE)*	*2003-4 (BE)*
Secretariat	3.24 (0.26)	3.37 (0.24)
DMSRHS	254.23(20.11) 13.40*	267.96 (19.41)
DME	389.04(30.77) 9.78*	461.99 (33.47)
DPH	420.45(33.26) 5*	500.59 (36.26)
Directorate of Family Welfare	114.45 (9.01)	67.28 (4.87)
Directorate of Drug Control	4.59 (0.36)	5.16 (0.37)
Directorate of Indian Medicine and Homeopathy	46.60 (3.68)	52.29 (3.78)
Directorate of TN State Health Transport	8.17 (0.65)	8.54 (0.62)
DANIDA	6.39 (0.51)	1.06 (0.077)
Reproductive Child Health	16.85 (1.33)	11.99 (0.87)
Total	1264.05	1380.28

Notes: Figures within parentheses indicate the percentage to the total.
* Indicates the percentage of funds allocated for drugs by the directorates. RE and BE refer to the revised and budget estimates respectively.

Source: Demand for grant, demand no. 18, Department of Health and Family Welfare, 2003-4, Tamil Nadu government, Budget publication no. 18.

Directorate of Medical Education (DME), Directorate of Public Health (DPH) and Directorate of Medical Services (DMS). In 2002-3, out of the total allocation of Rs. 1,264 crore for health, allocation towards medicines accounted for Rs. 93.09 crore or 7.36 per cent. Allocation for medicine works out to be 13.40, 9.80, and 5 per cent for DMS, DME and DPH, respectively, of their budget. The three directorates pass on 90 per cent of the budget meant for the purchase of drugs to TNMSC. Table 4.2 provides this data. TNMSC uses this amount to pay the suppliers. The remaining 10 per cent is retained with the directorates to purchase any drug outside the list, but considered essential. There is an application form in the TNMSC drug list, which the doctors can utilize to suggest inclusion or exclusion of a drug. Depending on the number of such applications TNMSC takes decision. TNMSC charges 0.50 per cent of each transaction as service charge as against the permitted 5 per cent. This is used for maintaining the office and the warehouse infrastructure.

SELECTION OF SUPPLIERS

TNMSC has laid strict and elaborate procedures to identify suppliers for its drug procurement to ensure uninterrupted and quality supply since making medicines available at the govern-

TABLE 4.2: ALLOCATION OF BUDGET TO TNMSC FOR THE PURCHASE OF DRUGS AND SURGICALS

(*Rs. in crores*)

Year *1*	*DME* *2*	*DMS* *3*	*DPH** *4*	*Total*
1995-6	26.07	27.74	10.68	64.49
1996-7	29.47	31.44	13.39	74.30
1997-8	32.32	33.19	14.28	79.79
1998-9	33.54	35.52	16.85	85.91
1999-00	34.76	32.53	18.16	85.45
2000-1	36.79	35.53	21.62	93.94
2001-2	37.77	35.73	18.03	91.53
2002-3	38.02	34.04	21.03	93.09

Note: *includes medicines to PHCs and the public health schemes.
Source: TNMSC.

ment health institutions is the primary purpose of setting up this organization. Accordingly rules and regulations are laid out. The first and foremost condition is that only manufacturers and direct importers of medicines can participate in the tender process. TNMSC invites tender by advertising in various dailies, pharmaceutical newspapers and on its own website. Tender document consists of Cover A and Cover B. The salient features of Cover A are: (a) the manufacturer should have license for the product quoted (loan licensing is not allowed) and should be manufacturing in his own premises; (b) the said company should have a minimum turnover of Rs. 35 lakh and the manufacturer should have market standing for the drug issued for a minimum period of three years; (c) the company should have the 'Good Manufacturing Practice' certificate issued by the state government authorities and should not have suffered any legal conviction cases. If the tender committee is satisfied with details provided in Cover A, then a technical team visits the unit (without prior notice to the unit) to assert the facts stated in the tender to assert the company's production capacity. On the basis of recommendation from the team, samples of drugs are obtained from the unit and sent for quality checks. On positive recommendation from the quality control department, those manufacturers who satisfy the entire criterion mentioned in Cover A are invited for the opening of Cover B. These manufacturers are asked to bring sufficient number of photocopies of their quoted prices and a floppy containing the prices of the products tendered by them. While photocopies are distributed to all those who are present in the tender process, the prices are simultaneously displayed on a huge screen. This method apparently helps in keeping the system transparent since every bidder gets to know the price bid by the other. Obviously, the one who has quoted the lowest price (called as L1) gets the tender. But if there are a couple of manufacturers whose prices are close to the L1 rates, they are asked to match the price of L1, and the entire purchase order is distributed accordingly. Price fixed during the tender process holds good for the whole year[4] and cannot be changed. In the whole tender process, there is neither any special preference for SSIs nor for public sector units.[5] Interestingly, suppliers in the current year do not automatically become eligible to supply the next year. They will have to go through the same procedures but for the inspection of units. This ensures transparency in the operation.

The other interesting feature is that, once the order is placed, the selected supplier should start supplying within 30 days of the contract and complete the same within/on the 60th day. A late delivery fee of 1.50 per cent of the entire purchase order is levied on the supplier, if the supplies are delayed even by a day. The supplier will have to send the supplies directly to the designated drug warehouses. On receipt of the drugs, the warehouse issues a Material Received Certificate (MRC) to the TNMSC office. A certain quantity of drugs drawn from each batch is sent for quality control to designated laboratories all over the country again selected through the tender process. This is done in spite of the fact that suppliers send their goods with QC certificate, a testimony that the products were checked before they were sent. Quality control takes about two weeks to test tablets and capsules and three weeks to test injections. Cold storage items are not sent for quality checks because appropriate temperature will have to be maintained throughout their journey. Surgical instruments and sutures are selected based on the recommendation of experts. Drug distribution takes place only after the receipt of report from the QC. If negative reports are received on a particular product, then that product is sent for QC to another laboratory. If it fails in the second time also, then the entire batch is sent back to the supplier, who will have to supply fresh stocks. If this happens twice, then the supplier is blacklisted. From May 2003, warehouses have been advised not to send samples of the same batch for testing, if samples of a particular batch have already been sent for QC. Similarly, if the QC passes a drug of a particular batch, then other warehouses can also start distributing. TNMSC makes payment to the supplier only after the report from quality control is received. An automated cheque clearance system of payment to the suppliers also helps in maintaining the transparency of the system.

Storage and Distribution of Drugs

In order to store the drugs, 24 warehouses have been built in 23 of the total 29 districts (Chennai has two warehouses, also see

Figure 4.4 for District Map of Tamil Nadu). All the warehouses are of uniform design and structure. Of the 24 warehouses, 2 were built with DANIDA's assistance and 11 were built with World Bank loan and the state government built the rest. All the warehouses except the one at Sivaganga are housed in their own building. Electronic trolleys are also available for facilitating loading the medicines in order within the warehouse. The total staff at the warehouse consists of two pharmacists (who are on deputation from government hospitals) one data entry operator (on a consolidated pay) and two helpers (outsourced) who help in the loading and unloading operations. These two are also not regular employees of the corporation. The pharmacists have been trained in drug handling, storage and distribution.

FIGURE 4.4: DISTRICT MAP OF TAMIL NADU

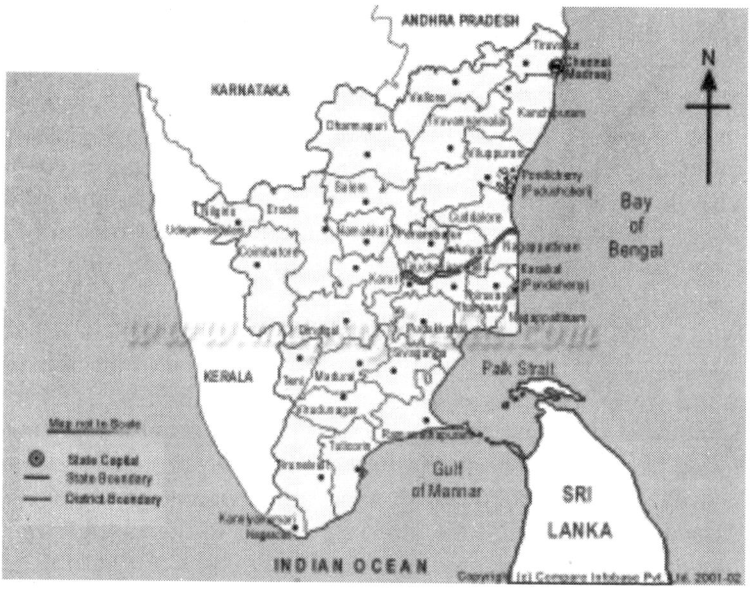

Note: TNMSC warehouses are in Kanchipuram, Vellore, Thiruvannamalai, Cuddalore, Dharmapuri, Salem, Erode, Coimbatore, Nilgiris, Tiruchirapalli, Pudukkottai, Dindugul, Madurai, Virudhunagar, Sivaganga, Ramanathapuram, Tirunelveli, Tuticorin, Nagercoil, Thanjavur, Villupuram, Chennai and Nagapattinam.

The decision of the TN government to have its own warehouses to handle the medicines is an important aspect in the distribution of the drugs. Since the warehouses are situated in different districts, health institutions in a particular district can draw their stock from the warehouse in that district. Taking into account factors like stock in hand, demand from various institutions and the stock that is to arrive, TNMSC places the purchase order worth a few months stock with the suppliers who supply directly to the warehouses. By getting the stock directly to the warehouse, the difficulty faced in the Central Medical Stores office of distributing to the different health institutes is avoided.

On arrival, appropriate entries are made in the computer about the stock that has arrived on that day, pending stock, quantity received until then, drugs distributed to different institutions, expiry date of the drug of different batches, stock at the warehouse and drugs that are sent for QC checks. These help the Chennai office in updating the stock position and also transferring drugs from one place to another in case of need. To make the system foolproof, TNMSC has stipulated the system of receiving the information by courier everyday. The warehouses are required to maintain a three-month stock and a safety limit of one-month stock.

All the institutions are provided with two passbooks valid for one accounting year, of which one is retained with the institution and the other with the warehouse, wherein the budget for that institution is mentioned. Budget for each institution is arrived at looking at the patient inflow and outflow in a particular year, disease pattern and drugs consumed. All the institutions in a particular district draw their drug stock from the warehouse of that district on their designated day. While teaching medical institutions draw their stock every month, PHCs draw their stock once in three months. TNMSC arranges transport for institutions, which draw drugs worth more than Rs. 1 crore. Each institution submits an indent form which indicates particulars like the stock in hand at the institution, stock required, stock supplied, batch number, expiry date, cost of the drug and so on. Appropriate entries are made in the passbooks and in the computer, which helps in tracing the movement of the drugs for the TNMSC and in monitoring over and underutilization of budget allocation for the different district health authorities. While the hospitals can indent any drug from the list, the list of drugs meant for PHCs is limited to 54 essential drugs.

PRICES OF THE DRUGS

One important outcome of this type of pooled procurement is that of low prices of drugs. TNMSC has been able to procure medicines at a low price and has also been able to maintain the price line for many years. Tables 4.3-4.5 show that: (a) adoption of EDL and proper procurement procedure have resulted in enormous reduction in the price paid for selected medicines compared to the earlier regime; (b) with continued vigilance and emphasis, TNMSC procures medicines at competitive prices and at the same time of good quality and (c) the impressive price difference between drugs bought in generic name and brand names because of rationalization of the drug expenditure. All these emphasize that substantial reduction in the government's drug expenditure can be made if only they are rationally prioritized and spent. The point that is emphasised here is that drugs being an important cost in the illness episode of consumers, any savings made in this arena can be used to widen the reach of public utilities to more consumers or in the form of more facilities.

TABLE 4.3: COMPARISON OF PRICES BEFORE AND AFTER TNMSC

(*in Rs.*)

Year/ Drug	*Pyrazinamide Tablet 10 × 10*	*Cloxacillin Capsule 10 × 10*	*Norfloxacin Tablet 10 × 10*	*Atenolol Tablet 10 × 10*	*Ciprofloxacin Tablet 10 × 10*
1992-4	135.00	158.25	290.00	117.12	525.00
2003-5	51.88	58.48	54.55	12.00	82.00

Source: TNMSC.

TABLE 4.4: PRICES OF DRUGS PURCHASED BY TNMSC, 1998-2003

(*in Rs.*)

Year/ Drug	*Paraceta-mol Tablet 10 × 10*	*Cotrima-xazole Tablet 10 × 10*	*Cephat-axime Sodium Inject*	*Ciprof-loxacin Injection 100ml ffs*	*Cipro-floaxacin Tablets 10 × 10*	*Ranitidine Tablets 10 × 10*
1998-9	13.14	31.0	8.31	8.00	168.00	31.20
1999-2000	11.95	27.85	5.67	7.50	129.60	28.00
2000-1	11.50	27.30	5.24	7.20	99.90	26.00
2001-2	11.42	27.82	5.08	6.75	93.03	23.90
2002-3	11.24	27.82	4.94	6.74	88.00	22.34
2003-5	12.40	24.88	4.41	6.41	82.00	22.05

Source: TNMSC.

TABLE 4.5: COMPARISON OF TNMSC AND MARKET PRICES

Product	*Unit of Drug*	*TNMSC Price*	*Market Price*
Aspirin Tab IP	10×10 tabs	12.17	44.42 (Ecosprin)
Paracetamol Tab IP	10×10 tabs	11.69	68.00 (Fapanil)
Paracetamol Syrup IP	60 ml	3.20	19.57 (Calpol)
Co-Trimoxazole Oral Suspension IP	50 ml	4.06	10.0 (Septran)
Co. Trimoxazole Tab IP	10×10	28.37	63.20 (Septran)
Metronidaxole Tab IP	10×10	13.21	36.50 (Flagyl)
Amoxcycilin Cap IP	10×10	78.47	366.66 (Novamax)
Erythromycin State Oral Suspension	40 ml	8.76	25.27* (60 ml) (Novamax)
Tetanus Toxoid Injection IP	5 ml	6.93	

Anti-Rabies Vaccine	3 ml	18.00	294.0 (Aventis)
Ciprofloxacin Inj IP	100 ml	7.00	46.89 (Cifran)
Gentamycin Eye and Ear Drops BP	5 ml	3.56	7.51 (Gentics)
Atenolol Tab IP	14×10	15.26	310.0 (Tenormin)
Ibuprofen Tab IP	10×10	13.10	55.55 (Brufen)

Note: Both TNMSC and market prices are inclusive of taxes.
Source: TNMSC L1 prices for the year 2002-3 provided by TNMSC, and the market prices are the prevailing brand prices collected from a medical shop in Chennai in June 2003.

5. IMPACT OF ADOPTING A RATIONAL DRUG APPROACH

As a result of the appropriate planning and pooled procurement procedures, TNMSC was able to show a savings of Rs. 32 crores in the first year of operation itself. With such savings made, now TNMSC has widened its activities to purchase of equipment to improve the technology available with the public hospitals, which makes them technologically comparable with the private sector hospitals. A total of 35 CT scan machines have been bought at a total cost of Rs. 25 crore and have been installed in the district headquarters hospitals, which are available to the general public on payment of a fee which depends on the economic criteria. Two MRI scans have also been installed in two government hospitals in Chennai and Madurai.

Though it would have been ideal to compare TN's expenditure on drugs with that of a state which has not adopted a rational drug list, in the absence of such data, we have attempted to compare the average medical expenditure per treated ailment for various states provided by the NSS for the year 1995-6 (Table 4.6). Here the medical expenditure includes expenditure on items like medicines, bandages, plaster, etc., fees paid for medical and para-medical services, charges for diagnostic tests, charges for operation therapies, charges for ambulance, cost of oxygen and blood, etc. These data show that the various states but for TN have invariably spent large amounts of financial

TABLE 4.6: AVERAGE MEDICAL EXPENDITURE PER TREATED AILMENT IN 1995-6 (GOVERNMENT SOURCE)

States	*Rural*	*Urban*
Andhra Pradesh	44	67
Assam	145	171
Bihar	169	65
Gujarat	61	117
Haryana	198	636
Karnataka	61	120
Kerala	85	78
Madhya pradesh	94	477
Maharashtra	73	91
Orissa	118	128
Punjab	137	201
Rajasthan	181	157
Tamil Nadu	10	23
Uttar Pradesh	363	228
West Bengal	157	72
All India	110	146

Source: Table 1.19, *Sarvekshana*, vol. 23, no. 3, January-March 2000.

resources on medicines. In fact, TN has spent the least compared to the other states, which may be attributed to the reforms introduced in the drug delivery system of TN.

6. REPLICABILITY OF TNMSC MODEL

The reform measures introduced by TN through TNMSC are highly localized. If such advantages have to be widespread all the state governments should adopt similar systems. Allured by the functioning of TNMSC, several state governments have come and studied the system. TNMSC itself has provided consultancy services to the state governments of Rajasthan, Karnataka, Gujarat, Orissa, Delhi and Andhra Pradesh. Andhra Pradesh has set up an agency like TNMSC and Orissa too has put the system in practice. But some state governments have not found any headway in this. Then what makes the system work in Tamil Nadu? The following paragraphs provide some explanation to this question.

The entire process adopted to streamline drug supplies can be broadly called as an effective implementation of drug policy in the state. While setting up of the TNMSC can be considered as the right type of government intervention, the activities undertaken by TNMSC can be classified as an Innovative Administrative Reform (IAR). We call it an IAR because these are reform measures thought over and introduced by the government to correct an existing government system of purchase of medicines that was plagued by several problems. Taking appropriate measures and placing them properly have rectified these problems. In a nutshell, elements like adoption of an essential rational drug list and efficient administration of the procurement and distribution procedures through an autonomous agency and most importantly, political support has resulted in the success of the model. Political support is essential to tackle the opposition that could arise from the transfer or reduction of financial powers that institutions hold in the purchase of medicines and the pharmaceutical industry, which may oppose purchase of generic drugs.

It should be mentioned that since the government planned the intervention and the team of bureaucrats and technocrats put the system in practice by laying strong principles in such a way that even a new government with a different ideology does not affect the functioning of the system. Also, it should be emphasized that the successive governments in TN have been only 'pro poor'. So any programme that directly benefits the poor and provides political mileage will only be continued. Further, in the case of TNMSC, setting up of the corporation or planning the purchase and distribution of drugs did not require any separate budget allocation and thus no financial burden on the state. All it required was to reallocate the budget and spend it rationally, through a corporation created exclusively for this purpose.

However, it can be argued that there are hundreds of corporations elsewhere set up exclusively for the development or sustainability of a particular sector, that are functioning below their capacity. What makes TNMSC a distinct entity is that this corporation works as an autonomous body within the overall framework of the state government. As a corporation, its overheads are limited because of its limited manpower and outsourcing of most employees. Secondly, as an autonomous organization which is in charge of purchase of drugs and equipment its procedures and operations are transparent.

The other important factor is the adoption of a rational drug list. This list identifies the important drugs that have to be bought, so a sizeable percentage of wastage of expenditure is controlled at this point itself. Further, the freedom given to the institutions for purchase is limited to 10 per cent only and centralized purchase covers 90 per cent of the budget, which again restricts pilferage. In some other states where a state formulary exists, shortages are often the case since; the percentage of procurement with the institution is high and varies from 50 to 90 per cent, allowing wastages, pilferages and also favouritism, leading to rent-seeking behaviour. Critics may argue that a centralized purchase could also lead to pilferages. However, as long as the procedures and guidelines remain transparent, the system will be effective. It should also be noted that after TNMSC started its operations, technology available in public hospitals has also started improving. While it would be extremely difficult to extend the rational drug approach to the private sector, any government with the political will and commitment can implement this model in its public utilities and also in the government funded/aided voluntary organizations.

CONCLUSION

The perspective on the role of government in providing health ranges from social welfare approach, public-private partnership to user-fee based market economy approach. However, if majority of the population does not have any health cover and if people below poverty line are dependent on the government health care system then a social welfare approach is desirable. One of the objectives of the Pharmaceutical Policy 2002 of the Government of India is to ensure abundant availability of good quality essential medicines of mass consumption at reasonable prices to the general public. It is a known fact that in India, private health expenditure is very high since people without medical cover bear their own expenditure. From this percentage of population, though it can be debated about the number of people accessing the government health care facilities, the NSS survey (1995-6) observes that households Below the Poverty Line (BPL) rely substantially on public services for all categories of health services and their utilization is significantly more than that by households above the poverty line (Sarveskshana, 2000). This combined with the fact that cost of medicines account for substantial share in the treatment of an ailment and considering the socio-economic cost of illness, the TN model only emphasizes that governments should strengthen the access to medicines in its health institutions.

TNMSC type of autonomous agencies may incur difficulties if the authorities working in such agencies are political appointees and do not have authority to take independent decisions, which is why many state governments are not able to adopt such a system. The TN model will continue to be successful as long as the systems remain transparent and uninterrupted medical supplies are ensured. The model ensures that the system is in place. To actually transform the availability of medicines in the government health care system into positive health outcome of people depends on further reforms.

NOTES

1. In this paper, the terms drugs and medicines have been used interchangeably.
2. The details of the drug supply models discussed here have been drawn from *Essential Drugs Monitor*, nos. 25 & 26, 1998.
3. During 1986-8, DANIDA was providing a kit of 15 essential medicines to the sub-centres in its area of operation. Though found to be useful, it was not operationalized or adopted for other health centres.
4. These prices are also posted in the TNMSC website and available at www.tnmsc.com.
5. There was a recent news item which said that with the change in the top officials in TNMSC, SSIs again want to take up their case and ensure that preference is given to them in the selection of suppliers.

REFERENCES

Dreze, Jean and Amartya Sen, *India Economic Development and Social Opportunity*, New Delhi: Oxford University Press, 1995.

Duggal, Ravi, Sunil Nandraj and Asha Vadair, 'Health Expenditures Across States, Parts I and II', *Economic and Political Weekly*, vol. 30, no. 15, 1995, pp. 834-44, vol. 30, no. 16, pp. 901-8.

Dukes, Graham, and Paula Munderi, 'Interim Report of Taskforce 5: Working Group on Access to Essential Medicines', 2004, available at http://www.unmillenniumproject.org/documents/tf5ateminterim.pdf.

'Drug Supply Choices: What Works Best?', *Essential Drugs Monitor*, nos. 25 & 26, Geneva: World Health Organization, 1998.

Essential Drugs Monitor, Geneva: World Health Organization, various issues.

Guhan, S. 'Social Security Initiatives in Tamil Nadu 1989', Working Paper No. 96, Chennai: Madras Institute of Development Studies, 1989.

———, 'Social Expenditure in the Union Budget–1991-1996', *Economic and Political Weekly*, vol. 30, nos.18 & 19, 6-13 May 1995.

Lalitha, N. 'Access to Medicines: Initiatives in Policy Making and Delivery of Drugs: A Case Study of Tamil Nadu', a report submitted to the World Bank, 2003.

Mahal, Ajay. 'The Distribution of Public Health Subsidies in India', in Abdo Yazdeek and David Peters, eds., *Health Policy Research in South Asia: Building Capacity for Reform*, Washington D.C.: World Bank, 2003.

Poornalingam, R. 'Drug Management in the Government Sector: The Tamil Nadu Model', *Essential Drug Monitor*, no. 21, Geneva: World Health Organization, 1996.

———, 'Drug Management in the Government Sector: The Tamil Nadu Model', Ranjit Roy Choudhury, ed., *International Experience in Rational Use of Drugs*, vol. 3, Thailand: The College of Public Health, Chulalongkorn University, Bangkok, 1998, pp. 97-120.

Prabhu, K. Seeta, *Economic Reform and Social Sector Development: A Study of Two Indian States*, New Delhi: Sage Publications, 2001.

Sarvekshana, 'A Note on Morbidity and Treatment of Ailments', NSS 52nd Round (July 1995-June 1996), vol. 23, no. 3, January-March 2007.

CHAPTER 5

Health Sector Reforms in Orissa: Some Experiences

SUBRATA KUNDU

THE PROBLEM

The term *health sector reforms* is a contested category around the world. It is being interpreted as a phenomenon of the 1980s and 1990s. Various articles dealing with health sector reforms hardly ever define the term and many of them just describe the existing health care services structure in different countries, in a topic claiming to deal with health sector reforms.[1] What most of these writings have done is to highlight the recent changes in the health care structure along with efforts towards privatization of health care in different countries of the world. Due to this definitional confusion, almost any major change in the health services sector either at a national or international level has been termed as health sector reforms.[2] Thus initiation of a new programme or even a change in approach in an existing programme like Reproductive and Child Health (RCH) has been termed as a reform initiative. Writing a paper or editing a volume without defining the term does not help much either for advancement of a theory or for a policy decision. This aspect was well recognized in a workshop held at Delhi's India International Centre by the Ministry of Health and Family Welfare in the year 2003.[3]

In this paper we will be using the definition of reform keeping in view the various initiatives for private participation taken by different countries in the world as well as from the Indian and in particular the Orissa experience. We can define health sector reforms as any initiative by the state, which tries to reduce the role of government in health services sector while creating an atmosphere for a larger role for the private sector. Before elaborating on this definition it is important to make it clear that this does not claim to explain all the changes happening in the health care sector in recent times nor does it try to explain all the policy initiatives taken by the different governments around the world with regard to the health sector. However, this definition captures the dominant trend being introduced in the health sector in India and abroad, beginning with the decade of 1980s, which has the potential of affecting the totality of the health sector in the long run.

Traditionally, health has been seen as a domain of the government even in countries which followed a liberal capitalist model of development. However, with the oil shock of the 1970s many of the governments in the world faced fiscal crisis. Along with this the collapse of the Soviet Union created an atmosphere where liberal capitalist model was seen as the only model of economic development.[4] In this model the private sector and the market forces play a dominant role with the State acting as a facilitator. The assumption is that market has its own rationality and in the long run will benefit, even though at the initial stage there will be 'hardships'. This argument has also been extended to the health services sector. Now health is seen as an individual responsibility. After the 1990s it has been seen that governments around the world have been increasing the scope for private participation in the health services sector. The scope of private participation may vary from one country to another; it may be on a small or large scale but it is redefining the concept of health. Since this private participation is happening in an era when the market plays a dominant role in the process of economic growth, any kind of control by the State is seen or perceived negatively.

But those who extend this logic to the health services sector forget that one has to remain alive to face the hardships of market interventions. If somebody is suffering from a particular disease and he or she does not have the capacity to pay for its treatment, than that person cannot postpone his or her disease for a future date! Therefore idea of giving the responsibility of 'health' to an individual in an iniquitous world falls to its own logic.

In the case of India though reforms have been defined in various ways, the principal factor which has brought about structural changes in health care services in various states has been the initiative of the World Bank. This is not to deny that in some states like Orissa organizations like the DFID of UK and the European Commission do play an important role in the reform initiatives in the health sector.

The document which the path for increasing the role of the private sector in India was the World Bank document titled *Investing in Health* published in 1993.[5] Here an argument was advanced that over the years the central role of the State in the health sector has not achieved the desired goals of improvement in the health status of the population. It has spent money where it was least required, like the tertiary sector while areas where most of the resources should have gone like the primary sector, have been neglected the most. Hence a case was made that to increase the 'efficiency' and 'effectiveness' of the health care services the government should focus on primary-level care while giving most of the responsibilities for secondary- and tertiary-level care to the private sector.[6]

These reform initiatives have to be seen in the larger context of economic liberalization in India in the 1990s and the movement of different countries around the world towards a liberal capitalist model of economic development after the collapse of communism in the former USSR. Communist China liberalized its economy in the late 1970s. Thus major powers in the world and most of the countries except Cuba have accepted the liberal capitalist model of economic development where the private sector and the market forces are playing the dominant role and the State is trying to facilitate this process through favourable legislation and playing the role of a regulator to promote fair competition among the various private players. Along with economic liberalization many developed and developing countries have allowed increasing role for the private sector in health care. This is the trend in the UK, USA, China, Canada, Australia and many of the countries of Europe where the private sector is playing a dominant role in health care provisioning.[7]

Health along with education has been seen as a primary responsibility of the government in different countries of Europe, Russia, China, and India. However the economic liberalization of the early eighties and increasing economic interdependence of countries has shaken the rationales of social security. The collapse of communism and the embracing of market economy by large countries like China and India have led to a belief in one model of development. In this framework an individual is held responsible for his or her social security.

The reform measures in the health sector are evaluated in terms of 'efficiency' and 'effectiveness', which are also the criteria for measuring economic success.[8] With the increasing privatization of health care in various countries the cost of care has also increased significantly. Earlier studies have shown that the poor and the rich have unequal access to health care and hence utilization pattern varies among them. As a result the poor have more disease burden and bear the major chunk of mortality in a given population.[9] With the process of globalization, where there is increasing flow of goods, people, technology and ideas, inequalities have also increased. While some countries have gained others are the losers and within different countries a certain section of population has only benefited out of this process. When the health sector is privatized in this scenario it raises serious issues about universal access and utilization of health care services.

Privatization of health care has a tendency towards increasing cost of care and as a result a vast section of population does not get an opportunity for life-saving drugs or to be able to afford the cost of care. This phenomenon can be observed in the case of USA, where many observers have documented the increasing cost of care. In the case of China, which had developed a vast health care network in its rural areas, the scenario is changing very fast. While before the economic reforms in the late 1970s access to health care was almost universal, after the reforms the rural networks are almost crumbling and the cost of care has also been increasing. This phenomenon can also be observed in countries like the UK and Canada. If one observes the evolution of health care services of these four countries, one can see the emergence of a pattern. In all these countries the argument for economic reforms has also been extended to health sector reform. The measurement of success in the health sector is also the same as the broad economic field, namely 'efficiency', 'effectiveness' and so on. The inherent assumptions of the liberal economy that the market in the long run will ensure access to all are also extended to the field of health care. This has serious repercussions, for the initial 'hardship' generated by the market mechanism will ensure that the vast sections of the poor remain out of the purview of essential health care services.

Studies have also shown that increasing role of private sector tends to promote the curative aspect of care.[10] As private participation in health care is no different from its involvement in any other field, the primary aim is to generate profit. Hence private hospitals tend to concentrate in developed regions and on specialized areas of care. The increasing focus on curative aspect generates a belief that a disease is located in an individual body and the larger factors like social, economic and political issues are insignificant or they play a very minor role. This excessive focus on curative aspect also neglects the importance of preventive measures, which is a very important aspect of public health.[11]

Areas like health and education cannot be left to the private sector. Even the World Bank, which had earlier been advocating for lesser role for the government in health care, has revised its stand in recent years.[12]

Using the above theoretical frame this paper makes an attempt to explain the reform initiatives being taken by the state government in Orissa in the health services sector. Before proceeding further let us look at the socio-economic background of the state against which the health services structure is functioning.

SOCIO-ECONOMIC BACKGROUND OF ORISSA

Orissa is situated in the eastern coast of India with a population of nearly four million people. The state is a predominantly agrarian society where most of its population lives in rural areas. According to the 2001 census the percentage of its total population living in urban areas is only 15 per cent. Orissa is one of the poorest states in India, nearly 48 per cent of its population lives below the poverty line.[13] Due to the predominance of agriculture the relationship among various sections of the society is feudal in character. As a result caste plays a dominant role in different aspects of society. The political power in the state has mostly been with the Karana and the Brahmins for generations. There are various cultural trends, which can be observed among the various sections of the society. Among these various trends the Jagannath cult or culture, which has grown through various generations, is the dominant cultural trend among the Oriyas.[14] With almost half of its population living below the poverty line and more than 40 per cent from Scheduled Castes (SC) and Scheduled Tribes (ST), it becomes very challenging for the state government to ensure access to health care for all.

Out of its total population 22 per cent are ST and 16 per cent are SC. These two sections constitute the bulk of the poor in Orissa and they live in remote and hilly areas. Almost 81 per cent of the SC/ST population are landless labourers with very little assets.[15] The large number of ST in the state also results in different understandings of notions of good health. This cultural difference is a significant barrier for promoting universal health care. As a result in tribal areas it has been seen in many cases that while health care infrastructure is available, utilization is very low. Women from these two groups suffer from disadvantages of income, caste and gender discrimination in every aspect of life.[16]

In 1997, Infant Mortality Rate (IMR) in Orissa was 97/1,000 live births (SRS) and Maternal Mortality Rate (MMR) was 437/1,00,000 live births (NFHS I). Malnutrition among women and children is still very high. NFHS II suggests that 48.50 per cent of adult women in Orissa suffer from malnutrition. This is highest proportion in India.[17]

EPIDEMIOLOGICAL SITUATION IN THE STATE

Communicable diseases like malaria, tuberculosis and leprosy continue to be major public health problems in the late twentieth century in Orissa apart from filariasis in the coastal districts. According to one estimate more than 60 per cent of the diseases prevalent in Orissa are water related. Communicable diseases like diarrhoea and dysentery, worm infections and typhoid are present throughout the year. The state still has the largest number of deaths due to malaria in India. Malnutrition continues to be a major public health concern. NFHS II shows that while 54 per cent of the children under the age 3 years are underweight, 44 per cent are stunted (height/age) and 24 per cent are wasted (weight/height).

According to one estimate Non-Communicable Diseases (NCD) constitute 22 per cent of morbidity in the state and 16 per cent deaths are due to accident and injuries. Diabetes, cardio-vascular diseases, chronic bronchitis and asthma and mental illness constitute major NCDs in the state.[18] Apart from these, natural disasters like floods, droughts and cyclones in the coastal areas create havoc and increase morbidity and mortality among large sections of the population.

HEALTH CARE SERVICES STRUCTURE

Before proceeding further let us look at the organizational chart of health care services in Orissa. The Ministry of Health and Family Welfare is the nodal ministry for the health care services in the state. At the top of the hierarchy is the Minister of Health and Family Welfare. Under him is the principal secretary with four secretaries to assist him. They are in the hierarchical order of additional, joint, deputy and under secretaries. Apart from these four secretaries, the project director Orissa Health Systems Development Project (OHSDP) is of the rank of additional secretary. There are six technical directors who directly come under the principal secretary. These directors are mostly from the health care services cadre and hence have a medical background. The six directors are Director of Medical Education and Training (DMET), Director Health Services (DHS), Director Family Welfare, Director of State Institute of Health and Family Welfare (SIHFW), Director Drugs Control and Director of Indian Medicine and Homeopathy. Medical and nursing colleges comes under DMET. The health care services cadre comes under DHS. The Director of Family Welfare looks after the family welfare programme in the state.[19] The role of SIHFW has been to recruit and train staff for different health programmes in the state. It has recently been given the status of Regional Training Center to train health personnel from Orissa, Jharkhand and Chhattisgarh.[20] The Chief District Medical Officer (CDMO), who is in-charge of a district, comes directly under the control of DHS. Director Drugs Control is the nodal agency for checking the quality of drugs in the private sector in the state through its drugs inspectors. It also issues licenses to private health care sector in the state. At the district level ADMO Public Health, ADMO Medical and ADMO Family Welfare assist the CDMO. The CHCs and PHCs come under the control of CDMOs.[21]

UTILIZATION PATTERN

The 42nd and the 52nd rounds of NSS show that Orissa is a state where there is higher utilization of public sector health care services by both the poor and the rich. This is due to the larger presence of the government sector in health care in the state and also due to the absence of a strong private sector, unlike in the other states. At present Orissa have 158 CHCs, 1,349 PHCs and 5,927 sub-centres. There are in total 181 hospitals. This includes 3 medical college hospitals, 31 district headquarter hospitals, 21 sub-divisional hospitals and 126 other hospitals.[22] The absence of the private sector can be explained by the fact that Orissa is not a developed state. Most of its population lives in rural areas with low per capita income. Along with this almost 50 per cent of its population lives below the poverty line. In these circumstances there is very little incentive for the growth of the private sector in the state. As studies by Baru and others have shown, the private sector has a tendency to move to the developed areas or developed regions and it is purely guided by the profit motive. As a result it not only focuses on select geographical areas, it also provides a narrow range of services.[23]

Thus we saw that Orissa is a state where the government has played a dominant role over the years in terms of provisioning of health care services. To provide health care to the different sections of the population the health care services structure has also expanded in the state over the years. But there is still a lot be done. Field visit to different single-doctor PHCs showed that there was absence of doctors and often it were, the pharmacists who ran these institutions. Many of the PHCs and sub-centres were run in rented buildings. That means at the ground level these do not function at all.[24]

All over India it has always been difficult for the state governments to retain doctors in rural and remote areas where there is absence of proper transportation and communication and other infrastructure facilities. This problem is also there in Orissa but in an acute form. The major reason for this is that there is almost always political interference in postings and transfers and according to informed sources it has turned out to be a lucrative industry.[25] However, while those with connections do benefit from this system, it has demoralized doctors at every level. This has significant implications for delivery of health care at the periphery-level institutions. Many observers are of the opinion that the periphery-level institutions have almost 'collapsed'.[26] Hence a question arises as to how different national programmes perform under these circumstances? In this background let us see in what areas 'reforms' have been initiated and are they addressing any of these issues?

REFORM INITIATIVES

Two events are supposed to have started the reform initiatives in the state. One was the formation of a House Committee of State Legislature, which looked into different aspects like raising resources for the ailing health care sector, introduction of user charges in medical colleges and district hospitals and on the issue of abolition of private practice by government doctors. Another event was an evaluation by the UK development agency DFID about its earlier two projects in Orissa.[27] However, there was one institution, that played an important role in the health sector reforms in the state—the Orissa Health Systems Development Project (OHSDP). This is a World Bank-funded project for 'revamping' secondary- and tertiary-level institutions in the state. However, the single connecting thread to these separate events is the effort to privatize the health services sector in the state. For this to happen there was a wider atmosphere of economic reforms initiated in India and various fiscal measures adopted by the state government. This larger atmosphere in fact acted as a legitimizing authority for 'reform' measures being initiated in the health services sector in the state.[28] Now let us look at some of the reform initiatives taken in the state.[29]

Introduction of User Charges

This was introduced in 1997 in medical college hospitals, all district-level government hospitals and in the Capital Hospital. The idea was to generate some funds for maintenance of equipment and furniture in these institutions. User charges have been introduced for all except those below the poverty line. For which services or for which diagnostic categories users will be charged has been left for each institution to decide. For the district-level hospitals, the money collected through user charges is kept in a fund under the zilla swasthya samitis. After the 'successful' introduction of user fees at various district-level hospitals the Government of Orissa is trying to introduce it in the sub-divisional hospitals as well.

Creation of District Cadre for Paramedics

Earlier the paramedical staff were recruited by the state government and were assigned to different districts. However, the staffs from coastal areas were unhappy to be posted in western Orissa or in the interior parts. As most of the paramedics were and are female staff they found it difficult to stay away from their families. To address this situation the Government of Orissa created a district cadre of paramedics, where the paramedic has to be from the same district. However these staffs are now recruited on a contractual basis.

Privatizing Cleaning in Government Hospitals

Initially it was introduced in the hospital in Bhubaneswar and has been extended to three medical colleges and to some district hospitals. In these institutions the government is no longer recruiting new sweepers, however the old staff are retained and after their retirement no recruitment is done to fill these vacancies. Hence the idea is to give the cleaning aspect to the private sector.

MULTI-SKILLING OF HEALTH PERSONNEL

This reform measure was introduced to utilize the existing capacity of the lab technicians fully. Before the introduction of this new measure, a lab technician for TB used to look after only TB slides and not those of malaria or leprosy. This was thought to be a waste of human resources. It was also realized they it would be an unnecessary expenditure to recruit another technician for the same lab. Multi-spilling of health staff was introduced in 1998 all over the state. One of the purposes of this initiative was to *cut costs* and use the existing resources, in this case manpower, *effectively*.

Since this initiative talks about cutting costs and using resources effectively within the larger frame of fiscal austerity by the state government, it has been included as a reform initiative.

DRUGS REFORM

The driving force behind the drugs reforms was to cut costs and make available quality care to the people who utilize government health care services. The reform that was introduced in 1998 was the adoption of the Tamil Nadu model. The principal features of this reform are: central procurement of drugs, adoption of an essential drugs list from WHO and shifting from brand drugs to generic drugs. After the reform measures the drugs are purchased centrally through an open tendering system and distributed to the districts. It is to be remembered that the reform measures in this sector are applicable only for the government health care sector. This 'reform' measure is supposed to be one of the success stories in the state.

HANDING OVER PHCS TO NGOS

This was introduced on a pilot basis in 1997 to see whether the arrangement works out or not. In remote and difficult areas it has been difficult to manage the PHCs, as the medical officer-in-charge remains absent for most of the time. There is also the problem of maintaining the morale of the other staffs in these institutions. As a result the essential primary health care services were not available to the people in these areas. To address this the Government of Orissa came out with this idea. However the experience in this sector has not been positive and the experiment has been abandoned for the time being.

There are other measures which have been termed as 'reform' but have not been included here as 'reform'. Some of these measures are:

Petty Maintenance for Buildings at PHC Headquarters

Rs. 10,000 per year is given to the medical officer-in-charge at the PHC to spend for petty maintenance, at his or her discretion. This has not been included as a reform measure in this paper because it does not fulfil our definition of reform, which is looking at any element of private participation in it.

Mandatory Pre-PG Rural Service

Under this scheme any medical graduate aspiring for a PG degree must serve for one year in rural and remote areas after getting selected for a PG course. This was introduced to address the absence of doctors in rural and remote areas in periphery-level institutions like PHCs. However, this criterion also do not fulfil our criteria for reform as there is not element of private participation in it.

Internship Training for Medical Graduates

This scheme was introduced in the year 2000 to train medical graduates in Social and Preventive Medicine under the guidance of a CDMO. This new measure was introduced to give exposure to the medical students about how the periphery-level institutions like PHCs and CHCs function at the grassroots level. This revised course curriculum gives medical students comprehensive training.

Pancha Byadhi Chikitsa Scheme

The above term in Oriya means 'treatment for five diseases'. This scheme was introduced in 1999 and it had identified five diseases—leprosy, malaria, acute respiratory infections, scabies and diarrhoea. These would be treated free of cost at any government hospital and medicines would also be given free. This scheme was introduced after on epidemiological study found that these diseases were the major reasons for morbidity and mortality in the state. Again this was a public health initiative by the Government of Orissa to respond adequately to epidemiological challenges in the state but does not fulfil our criteria of reform.

Creation of Zilla Swasthya Samitis

Earlier there were different societies to manage different diseases like malaria, TB, and so on at the district level. Funds were also maintained separately. However, to improve the management of these societies, it was decided to amalgamate them and create a new society in its place with the district collector as the chairman and the CDMO as the secretary. This scheme was introduced in 1999. This scheme aims at making effective the district-level societies but here too there is not a single element of privatization and hence it has not been included as an element of reform in this paper.

The criteria of selection of different initiatives as reform or not has significant repercussions. For even the so-called 'drugs reform' cannot be fully accepted as a reform initiative. For, all the three new elements introduced in the drugs sector in Orissa, namely, central procurement of drugs, adoption of an essential list from the WHO and shifting from brand names to generic names, are basically measures aimed at improving the quality of drugs available at government institutions and reducing the cost of drugs purchased. Hence there is hardly any element of 'reform' according to our definition. However, this new drugs policy by the state government can be termed as a measure towards improving the system of drugs supply while ensuring quality drugs are being supplied to the public from a government health institution. These changes can at best be termed as revisions by a government department to improve its performance and to cater better to the needs of the public. However, terming these initiatives as 'reforms' is not appropriate.

Every system tries to respond to the new challenges that it faces in its day-to-day functioning. In due course of time many of its elements, which were created with a particular set of purposes in mind, are not able to respond to the new challenges and hence these elements need to be replaced by others which can cope with the new challenges in a better way. Those changes, which have been termed as reform, in fact, are an attempt to make the system respond to the new challenges. Terming them reform initiatives is problematic.

Conclusion

This paper has attempted to look at some of the 'reform' experiences being undertaken in the health services sector in the Indian state of Orissa. However, along with this an attempt was also made to define the term health sector reforms keeping in view the larger initiatives taken by countries around the world. The importance of defining a term before proceeding to elaborate about its various aspects is very important. The various books and articles claiming to deal with health sector reforms have hardly ever come out with a clear-cut definition of the term. On the other hand, due to this definitional confusion, any major change in the health services sector has been termed as a reform initiative. This has not at all helped in clarifying matters.

There are research papers which have documented the increasing role of the private sector in the health services sector across the world, but they have also included different initiatives by governments as a 'reform' initiative. For example, the change in the approach towards RCH has been termed as a reform initiative. The definition given in this paper tries to explain the dominant trend in the health services sector that is occurring around the world, which has the potential not only to change the way health has been understood but also for its capacity to include large sections of population from basic health care services.

This can be observed from the fact that those countries, which earlier had the state playing a dominant role in terms of financing and provisioning of health care, are increasingly giving a larger role to the private sector. The arguments for reforming the health sector come from the broader field of economic reform initiatives, which have an unquestioning faith in the rationality of market forces. It has been argued here that with increasing globalization, characterized by increasing economic interdependence between different countries and movement of information and people across borders, inequalities have also increased.[30] In this scenario the increasing role of private sector has far reaching consequences. With the notion of 'individual responsibility for health' and private participation, health is increasingly being viewed in terms of its curative aspect and in the process neglecting the crucial preventive aspect of it.

Country experiences from the US and China show that with the increasing role of private sector in health care, cost of care also tends to increase over the years. As a result it becomes difficult for the poorer sections of a country's population to access basic health care services.

Taking the Indian state of Orissa as a case study an attempt has been made to define the criteria of health sector reforms. It has been shown that the measures, which are seen as a reform initiative may not be reform at all but only a systemic change to respond to the existing situation in a better way. The experience of reforms from Orissa shows an increasing trend of private participation in health services sector and a conviction at different levels of the state government that the private sector has a larger role to play in the health services sector.[31]

NOTES

1. A. C. Twaddle, ed., *Health Care Reform Around the World*, Westport: Greenwood Publishing Group, 2002.
2. See for example Peter Berman, ed., *Health Sector Reform in Developing Countries: Making Health Development Sustainable*, Boston: Harvard School of Public Health, 1995.
3. Proceedings of Workshop on 'India's Health System: Role of Health Sector Reforms', 4-5 September 2003, India International Centre, New

Delhi. Bureau of Planning, Directorate General of Health Services, Ministry of Health and Family Welfare, Government of India, New Delhi.

4. R. Baru, *Private Health Sector in India*, New Delhi: Sage Publications, 1998.
5. World Bank, *World Development Report 1993: Investing in Health*, Washington D.C: World Bank, 1993.
6. Ibid.
7. Twaddle, op. cit.
8. See for example Dr. Baru's article in I. Qadeer, K. Sen and K.R. Nayar, eds., *Public Health and Poverty of Reforms: The South Asian Predicament*, New Delhi: Sage Publications, 2001.
9. T. McKeown, *Sociological Approach to the History of Medicine, Medical History and Medical Care: A Symposium of Perspectives*, London: Oxford University Press, 1971.
10. Baru, op. cit.
11. Debabar Banerji, *Poverty, Class and Health Culture in India*, vol. 1, New Delhi: Prachi Prakashan, 1982.
12. See *World Development Reports* of World Bank since early nineties.
13. *Census of India*, 2001.
14. Also see a book by Manoranjan Mohanty and Bijay Kumar Bahidar titled *Orissa Daridra Kahinki?* (Why Orissa is Poor?), published by Orissa Book Store, 1993.
15. *Census of India*, 1991.
16. *Orissa Vision 2010: A Health Strategy*, February 2003, Health and Family Welfare Department, Government of Orissa.
17. Ibid.
18. Ibid.
19. See Organogram of the health services structure of the state given in the official website of Health and Family Welfare Department, Government of Orissa.
20. This was known from interview with a certain official in SIHFW, Bhubaneswar.
21. See the Organogram again.
22. Data collected in the year 2005 from the Directorate of Health Services, Government of Orissa.
23. Ibid.
24. This was observed during field visits to PHCs and sub-centres in Orissa.
25. This was known through interaction with various officials at different levels of the Health Services Structure in the Government of Orissa.
26. Ibid.
27. Meena Gupta, *State Health System: Orissa*, November 2002, New Delhi: ICRIER.

28. Interview with a World Bank official in New Delhi in 2004.
29. These criteria of identifying reform measures are taken from Meena Gupta's paper, from *Orissa Vision 2010* document and with various interviews with donor agencies and the state government officials.
30. See *Human Development Reports* since 2000 to 2004 published annually by UNDP.
31. Observations from the fieldwork in Orissa in the year 2005.

CHAPTER 6

The Myth of the *Mitanin*: Political Constraints on Structural Reforms in Health Care in Chhattisgarh

BINAYAK SEN

Since the middle of 2002, the newly formed state of Chhattisgarh has been the locus of a statewide programme of structural reforms in the government health care system. This programme was designed to have had two broad components: one was the articulation and popularization of the right to health care through a process of selection, training, and activation of community-based women health workers called *mitanins*. The other broad component was the implementation of a series of fundamental changes in the health care infrastructure of the state. Despite promising achievements in the area of infrastructure development, due to structural problems in the way in which the entire programme has been implemented, the political core of the programme remains unrealized. This major programme illustrates the structural constraints contingent upon state-based interventions in health care in the absence of major political initiatives.

Chhattisgarh is one of the three newly formed states of the Indian Union, having been established on the 1 November 2000. Apart from the sex ratio, all demographic indicators impacting on the health of the people are to the disadvantage of the people of the state. Hunger-related deaths have been occurring in recent years with increasing frequency. Investigations into such events carried out by the Chhattisgarh People's Union for Civil Liberties (PUCL), in which we participated, have shown: (a) a large section of the affected communities do not have the purchasing power to access the targeted public distribution system; (b) supply of safe drinking water is simply not available to many such communities; (c) the government health care facilities remain inaccessible to such communities; (d) BMI studies have shown that the median BMI in such communities is below 18.50. Of all these factors we have deliberately concentrated our attention only on aspects relating to health care in the analysis hitherto.

Within this context, the Government of Chhattisgarh (GoC) in January 2002 initiated a series of consultations to design a comprehensive programme of change to bring about specific changes in the health care system in the state. It was agreed that funding assistance for this ambitious programme would come from the European Commission under their sector reform programme. Apart from senior health care functionaries in the state, senior bureaucrats, civil society administrators, and health activists participated in this intensive colloquium.

What came out of this consultation was a two-pronged strategy: on the one hand a programme for the state-wide selection, training and deployment of community health workers and the other hand there was a 15-point programme for bringing about fundamental changes in the health care system in the state. We will now consider each of the two aspects in greater detail.

COMMUNITY HEALTH WORKER PROGRAMME

The programme envisaged the selection, training and deployment of a statewide system of community health workers. These workers were supposed to have certain special characteristic:

a. All the workers were to be women. They would be known as *mitanins*. The use of this term, which denotes a culturally hallowed relationship, generated considerable opposition; what was finally agreed upon was a compromise.
b. All the women would be selected from within the communities that they would be serving through a process of consensus.
c. The communities in question would be self-defined hamlets rather then villages. In other words any group of families

regarding themselves as a community would define themselves as such and proceed to select a health worker for themselves. This provision was specifically designed to tie in with the concept of 'gram sabha' in the PESA.

d. Educational attainment would not be a constraint on selection.
e. None of the *mitanins* received any salary or allowance from the government in lieu of their services. This provision generated a prolonged debate, but was agreed to on the grounds that the *mitanin* should be a community representative rather than a government functionary. This provision did not preclude the payment of compensatory allowances during training or the provision of community-based subventions at a later stage of the programme.
f. The *mitanin* would perform certain technical functions by way of first contact care within the community, for which she would be specifically trained over a period of time. However, her main function would be to articulate the demand for health care within the community in the form of right to health care. A slogan was coined '*Swasthya Hamar Adhikar Hawe* (Health is our Right)'.

THE HEALTH SECTOR REFORM AGENDA

A national-level consultation in January 2002 identified a number of areas of the current health services provision which needed structural changes in state policy and practice, in laws, in programmes and institutions. The focus was mainly on strengthening community health systems, primary- and district-level health delivery systems, health surveillance and epidemic control. The areas of reform, which would go along with the programme, are detailed below.

The agreed reform agenda underlined the following objective with role of civil society partners specified:

1. *Community-based health services*

- Assisting in the finalization of the community-based health programme of the GOC (*mitanin scheme*).

- Assisting in designing a social mobilization campaign for popularizing the idea of 'people's health in people's hands' and creating effective demand for the programme.
- Assisting in designing the media and communications strategy and package for the programme.
- Assisting in developing operationalization details and implementation schedules for the *mitanin* programme.
- Assisting in developing all training modules and pedagogy for the *mitanin programme.*
- Assisting in monitoring and evaluation of the programme.
- Assisting in the coordination and logistics for the training programmes.

2. *Delegation and decentralization*

- Assist GOC in developing an autonomy package for: (a) integrated District Health and Family Welfare Agency (DHA), (b) hospitals, (c) programme managers at district levels and (d) PRIs and urban local bodies (ULBs).
- Planning of devolution of financial powers and other resources, specifically financial resources to PRIs and ULBs.
- Strengthening the system of transparency, the right to information and social audits.

3. *Strengthening health intelligence, surveillance, epidemiology and planning*

- Review of current systems of health intelligence and surveillance, and proposing reforms in integrating the *mitanin* scheme.
- Developing systems of village and district health plans, with community participation.
- Improving the quality, reliability and analysis of statistics.

4. *Control of epidemics*

- Improving community and primary health care systems for: (a) prevention, (b) early detection, (c) early intervention, (d) early prevention of morbidity and mortality because of epidemics.

5. Health problems of poor people

- Participatory studies of major health problems of rural and urban poor people.
- Participatory plans at local, district and state levels to overcome the health problems of poor people.

6. Capacity-building

- Assisting in identifying capacity-building needs and training packages for the DHA officials and hospital managers to enable them to perform their new role effectively.
- Assisting in identifying capacity-building needs and designing training packages for the PRIs, starting from the gram sabhas and ULBs to make devolution of powers to control government health institutions and services effective.
- Assisting in building capacities to utilize existing funds, draw budgets and plan interventions.
- Assisting in building capacities to develop accountable community mechanisms like social audits to effectively manage and monitor the local health department.

7. Rational drug use policy

- Develop a rational drug use policy for the state.
- Monitor the implementation of the rational drug use policy.
- Establish transparent systems for community monitoring of the implementation of this rational drug use policy.

8. Improving internal systems of the Department of Public Health

- Identifying internal systems which need reform.
- Proposing changes for identified areas of reform.

9. Workforce management and transfer policy

- Assisting in the development of a workforce management policy which is clear and transparent.

10. Drug distribution and logistics

- Assisting in identifying bottlenecks in the distribution and supply of drugs.
- Conduct a feasibility study to set up a parastatal organization for the distribution and logistics of drug supply across the state.
- Based on the recommendations of the study, suggest policy norms and guidelines to further extend the reach of the state drug distribution network.
- Monitor the implementation of the new drug distribution norms.

11. Uniform clinical treatment protocols

- Recommend standardized clinical protocols across the state at the primary, secondary and tertiary level.

12. Management Information System

- Assisting GOC in designing comprehensive computerized management information system for the health department from the *mitanin* up to the district level.
- Assisting GOC in the user-need analysis as well define outputs expected from the MIS across all levels.
- Assisting GOC in the process flow analysis of the department.
- Assisting GOC in feasibility of hardware platforms and software across all levels of users within the health department.
- Assisting GOC in the development of at least two websites: one for the *mitanin* programme and another for the health department of the GOC.

13. Decentralized laboratory services

- Assisting in developing low-cost diagnostic tools and systems for decentralizing laboratory services to the primary care level.
- Assisting in developing training packages for 'barefoot laboratory assistants' across the state.

14. Mainstreaming of Indian systems of medicine, especially tribal medicines into the state health system

- Studying feasibility of integrating some aspects of traditionally practiced tribal medicine in Chhattisgarh.

15. Drug resistance in malaria

- Studying the extent of drug resistance (to cholroquine) in selected areas of Chhattisgarh.
- Focusing on the incidence and prevalence of forest-fringe malaria in Chhattisgarh and recommending comprehensive treatment protocols for malaria.

The Formation of The State Advisory Committee

Taking on board these suggestions, the Department of Health and family Welfare, Government of Chhattisgarh, decided to formally collaborate with the leading NGOs of the state who were involved in health action and who had been part of this process. These partners included Rupantar, Jan Swasthya Sahayog, Zilla Saksharta Samiti (Durg) and Bharat Gyan Vigyan Samithi (Raigarh) and Ambikapur Health Society and Ramakrishna Mission. A high-powered State Advisory Committee (SAC) was formed by a government order. This committee was constituted with representatives of these NGOs, of senior state health officials and of representatives of funding agencies contributing to health sector development to monitor the progress of the reform process as well as provide inputs for the community health worker programme.

Formation of the State Health Resource Centre

To provide on-going support to the health sector reform and development process and to facilitate this massive community health worker programme Action-Aid was requested to set up a State Health Resource Centre (SHRC), fully supported by the Government of Chhattisgarh in order to make available high-quality human resource support for health services in

Chhattisgarh. The terms of reference for this state health resource centre was agreed upon and crystallized in the form of a Memorandum of Understanding signed between the country director, Action-Aid and the Secretary, health.

The MOV defines the SHRC as 'an additional technical capacity to the Department of Health and Family Welfare in designing the reform agenda for the transition from existing health services to community-based health services, developing operational guidelines for implementation of the reform programme, and arranging/providing on-going technical support to the District Health Administration and others managing implementation of this reform programme.'

We can briefly take stock of the achievements of the programme upto the year 2005, before turning to an analysis of the various ways in which the programme has fallen short of its original objectives.

ACHIEVEMENTS OF THE PROGRAMME

Almost 50,000 *mitanins* have now been selected and brought into the training process. They have been attending the training programmes held across the state. Many of them have been participating in village-level family health surveys. Their help and participation is also being sought in monitoring some of the functions of the ANM and other paramedical staff. Large numbers of them have been issued with *dawa petis* (medicine kits). We do not at the moment have any feedback about their ability to use the kits. They have also been issued referral slips with which to send patients to the peripheral health care units.

An essential drugs list has been evolved, and doctors trained in its rationale and use. An entirely new procedure for the purchase, stocking and distributing drugs of assured quality has been evolved and is slowly being put in place. A series of standard treatment protocols have also been developed, both at the medical and paramedical levels, and relevant in-service training have been organized. A major workforce study has been undertaken and its implications are currently under consideration. A series of publications have been put out by the SHRC, drawing upon in-house resources as well as the services of external consultants.

These include a series of six *mitanin* training booklets, a publication on the conceptual and operational aspects of the *mitanin* programme, the Chhattisgarh State Drug Formulatory, Standard Treatment Guidelines for medical officers and para-medical workers separately, a study of workforce management and HRD in the public health care system, and the proceedings of a malaria operations research workshop.

The enchanced quality of primary health care programme has also been taken up by the SHRC. The central purpose of the programme is to strengthen service delivery in the public health system, both in terms of utilization and in terms of quality.

The Government of Chhattisgarh has begun by strengthening health services in 32 blocks so that over the next three to five years the process could be repeated till all 146 blocks are covered.

After discussions, participatory goal setting was abandoned in favour of a focus on reducing maternal mortality by:

a. Ensuring 24 hour emergency obstetric care capability in the CHC.
b. Ensuring 24-hour institutional delivery capability in every sector PHC.
c. Ensuring good quality services at the sub-centre.

It is reasoned that if the gaps are closed in infrastructure, equipment, manpower and skills, sufficient to provide the above, and it in parallel organizational and motivational processes are addressed then not only care at delivery but service delivery in the public system as a whole in that block would be strengthened. In parallel many other bottlenecks like better location of facilities, a working referral system, integration with the *mitanin* system and multi-skilling of workers would be addressed.

Many of these achievements have been obtained in the face of determined opposition from the many vested interests threatened by these measures. However, as we shall show, despite these changes, the possibilities created thereby for equitable, accessible, effective, and humane health care systems remain unaltered in the main. While a detailed analysis would yield many factors responsible for this outcome, the three major factors that we have identified are:

a. The total destruction of the political character of the community health programme.
b. The already highly privatized nature of the health service infrastructure in Chhattisgarh.
c. The failure to make any attempt at administrative and financial devolution within this programme.

The critical assessment that follows discusses these issues in greater detail and elaborates on some examples of fundamental confusion that have bedevilled the programme.

CRITICAL ASSESSMENT

In its original formulation the programme was to have had a woman community health worker who would work in her community to articulate the right to health care and a slogan to this affect had been developed, as has been mentioned. It was not mere naivety that persuaded us to accept the possibility of such a demand being articulated from within a state-sponsored and -implemented process. In the initial consultation, the State protagonists had taken care to involve civil society partners who had been working in Chhattisgarh and elsewhere to articulate peoples' rights to health through a variety of approaches. The list of participants included Shaheed Hospital which had done pioneering work in developing a curative health programme in the context of the Chhattisgarh Mukti Morcha; Rupantar, which had extended the ideas developed through the Shaheed Hospital experience to a tribal land movement context and had considerable experience in a community health worker based health programme; Raigarh Ambikapur Health Association which combined community-based health insurance and service delivery through a chain of primary, secondary and tertiary health facilities; CEHAT which worked in health advocacy and community health worker training in Maharashtra; BGVS, which had experience of social mobilization and demand articulation for health and literacy. All the participating civil society organizations had been given a categorical assurance that there would be a one-year pilot phase when they would have the opportunity to put this new concept of the community health worker on the ground, free of government interference and that these pooled experiences would be the basis for the further elaboration of the concept of the community health worker in Chhattisgarh. The civil society partnership in the programme was also sought to be formalized through the establishment of the State Advisory Committee (SAC). However the SAC was quickly marginalized in the decision-making process, and in fact, SAC meetings have not been held at all for the last 12 months (August 2003 to July 2004). However, this assurance was breached early in the programme. Once the State Health Resource Centre (SHRC) was properly set up and the programme got properly into swing, performance indicators took over under the aegis of an agency that considered itself to be a 'para-statal body'.

Moreover, once the power elite in the government and outside it realized that the *mitanin* was a handy new source of patronage within the village, they quickly took over and occupied all the vacant spaces in the implementation of the programme. Within a year of the establishment of the new state, a very large number of new NGOs crawled out of the wall to serve as vehicles for the hegemonic aspirations of the existing elites. This nexus exerted great pressure to rapidly expand the programme. As a result of this expansion, the focus shifted away from the rights-based approach to one that concentrated on technical milestones. This destroyed whatever possibilities were left in the development of an approach based on a realization of the right to health care. The para-statal body, which quickly became a 'quasi-statal body' implemented this total perversion of the original concept of the *mitanin*.

The current government health care infrastructure in Chhattisgarh is already heavily privatized. All salaried doctors are allowed private practice, and with rare exceptions, devote a large part of the working day to this activity. Moreover with the widespread application of user fee for service, government hospitals and health centres are almost universally places where effective treatment only becomes available after money changes hands. BPL card holders are eligible for free treatment, but in a state were 40 per cent of the people are calorie deficient, only 25 per cent of the people have BPL cards by World Bank fiat. Moreover, in a situation where most people pay, free often means inferior. Such norms have worked themselves down the line. ANMs charge Rs. 500 for a normal delivery, Multipurpose Health Workers charge Rs. 100 for a glucose drip and so on.

Public investment in such a structure can only increase the lack of equity and accessibility. This is not a plea for less public investment, but only a realization of the fact that unless the back of this corrupt system is broken, piecemeal approches will not work. No such attempt has been made within the parameters of the present programme. On the other hand, while the total budget of the entire health sector reform programme over three years is Rs. 16 crore, until now only Rs. 8 crore have been spent. In contrast, in the overall health budget of the state, Rs. 12 crore, out of an annual budget of Rs. 400 crore have already been invested in a public-private partnership with Escorts Heart Hospital. The latter facility is housed in one wing of the Raipur Medical Collage, an institution built totally out of public funds.

By devolution, we do not mean leaving impoverished communities with the impossible task of generating their own resources but to the transfer of real resources and decision-making power to communities and their federations. The entire legal and institutional apparatus for such a process already existed in Chhattisgarh, a state over large areas of which Extension of Panchayat Act in the Fifth Scheduled Area (PESA) is in operation and where PRIs are almost a decade old. The structural reform programme nevertheless remains highly centralized, with real power being exercised by a tiny group of people—ministers, bureaucrats, senior doctor, administrators and a 'para-statal body'. The entire panchayati raj system has been bypassed in this process. The long-term political results of such an approach will be interesting indeed to watch.

The confusion about the role of the *mitanin* and who she represents mirrors many of the issues we have discussed earlier. In the original conceptualization, the *mitanin* was envisaged as a community representative, and the argument for not paying her a salary was based on this notion. As a matter of fact, the PRI interface with the *mitanin* was supposed to look into the issue of compensating her for the service. Yet, as the programme grew more and more target driven, the onus for monitoring fell on the health and SHRC bureaucracy; the SHRC annual report for 2003-4 articulates the monitoring structure as 'a monitoring cascade where every functionary *above* the Mitanin has one or two formats to fill' (emphasis added). This was expected to 'track every Mitanin performance and send up only such information as can be acted upon at that level'. It adds that all necessary formats for this were to be printed centrally, and that the SHRC together with the district collectors and CMOs was to tighten monitoring.

The two key concepts of public-private partnership and state-civil society partnership that form a large part of the sector reform discourse are called into question through the experience of health sector structural reforms in Chhattisgarh. In many circles the programme in Chhattisgarh has been hailed as a success story, particularly for its operationalization of these two aspects. Yet, our discussion has shown that important political prerequisites for the creation of a just, equitable, accessible, and effective health care system have not been met in this process.

A widespread articulation of the right to health care is not a mere utopian dream. It is a necessary part of any process of genuine structural reforms in the health care system. In its current formulation, a liberatory role for the community health worker remains a myth—the myth of the *mitanin*.

CHAPTER 7

User Fee in Public Health Care Institutions

ABUSALEH SHARIFF AND SUBRATA K. MONDAL

INTRODUCTION

With a population of more than a billion—the second largest in the world—India has created a vast infrastructure in the health sector. More interesting is the diversified socio-economic nature of its population. India accounts for 16 per cent of the world's population and 21 per cent of the world's global burden of diseases. In India public and private enterprises and NGOs extend health care services independently of each other. Expenditure on health services is largely the care seekers' liability. Urban and rural health reflect altogether different scenarios in the country. The rural people basically depend on public health care services, because private practice in remote areas is not lucrative to medical graduates. The backbone of rural health is the Primary Health Centre (PHC). The PHCs mainly provide preventive and promotive services and rudimentary curative care. Therefore for serious curative care rural folks depend on the Community Health Centres (CHC) or rural hospitals, which are usually situated in talukas. Going to a CHC involves expenditure, including cost of transportation and opportunity cost that they forego during the illness episode. The expenditure may also include purchase of medicines, which many times are not available in the CHCs and in many public hospitals. It is also true that many rural people find urban health care facilities (public or private) more effective because they get a wider range of services here than in a CHC or rural hospital (RH).

On the other side, urban health care scenario is altogether different. Urban people have two options—they can either wait for a long time to get even a small ailment treated in a busy urban hospital, or they can rush to private practitioners. Now the question of payment arises. Public health care services are usually free, at least for rural and poor people. In the late 1990s the Government of India introduced user fees for using public health care services in referral public hospitals. As per the stated policy, the Below Poverty Line (BPL) households are exempted from user charge payments. Therefore, rest of the care seekers purchase health services either from public or from private establishments. At present user fees have been introduced in all facilities at the district-level hospital and other higher level facilities. Although utilization of public curative services by the urban poor is far from satisfactory, the rural poor seem to suffer from twin disadvantages. They have to incur huge money in terms of transportation and other incidental expenses even to access free public services in towns and cities. It is, however, expected that the rural poor would not hesitate to pay little amounts to buy quality health facility if provided in their vicinity. Therefore, it is a case of introducing graded user fees in public hospitals to ensure quality services to the rural people. On the other hand, the escalating demands on the health care system are making services costly and efforts to increase use at the lower levels needs additional resources. Severe resource constraints have led policy makers to consider alternative sources of financing for public health care systems. Hospital user fee, i.e. to charge actual costs from users who can afford them out-of-pocket, is one of the alternatives for health financing. A well-designed and implemented user fee can mobilize additional resources from better-off groups which can in turn be used to improve services for poorer groups; a system which is now a cross-subsidization of the poor by the well-off. Such cost-sharing schemes can play a critical role in ensuring essential services to the needy. The National Health Policy 2002 recognizes the practical need for levying reasonable user-charges for certain secondary and tertiary public health care services, for those who can afford to pay. Since the latter half of the 1990s, user charges on public health care services have been initiated in several states in the country.

This paper describes key features of the user fee system in detail as two case studies, one undertaken in the state of Uttar Pradesh and another in Orissa. The paper also reflects upon the practical experience of the user fee system in nine hospitals or CHCs across eight states—Uttar Pradesh, Karnataka, Orissa, West Bengal, Rajasthan, Madhya Pradesh, Gujarat and Tamil Nadu. An assessment has been made of the problems and complexities inherent in maximizing the efficiency gains and minimizing the equity losses resulting from user fee.

It was possible to undertake an analysis of disaggregated budgetary and expenditure trends of the hospitals and match them with user profiles. It was also possible to attempt a demand analysis for facilities where user charge financing has been initiated. Non-availability of budgetary data, poor patient (IPD and OPD) record keeping and non-availability of gender disaggregated patients' profile made it difficult to conduct a precise appraisal. However, the data analysis does point to an urgent need to undertake highly focused studies across India, on the implementation and success of 'hospital user fee' system. The findings presented in the following sections are based on hospital records made available, visits to health institutions, and in-depth interviews with hospital and district officials.

USER CHARGES—A REALITY

User charges were introduced in different states at different points of time, except in Gujarat and Tamil Nadu where it has not been introduced. Karnataka was the first state to introduce user charges on hospital services in 1996, followed by Orissa in 1997, Madhya Pradesh in 1998, Uttar Pradesh in 2000 and West Bengal and Rajasthan in 2001. The basic form of user fee administration and broad categories of user charges were found to be more or less uniform across states. User charges were initiated at the issuance of a government order from the health secretary in each state, following which a hospital-level committee was constituted for the management of the user fee system. The government order specified the arrangements for the administration of the user fee system as well as guidelines under which user fee would be collected and spent. Under these guidelines provided by the government, the hospital authorities act as the decision-making body and exercise control over the expenditure of the revenue raised from user fee collections. Committees have been set up in each hospital and guidelines have been laid down to manage the fund. A state-level body is supposed to monitor the hospital-level committees.

The usage pattern of the funds collected is more or less uniform. The funds are to be utilized to improve the operations and maintenance of the hospitals and thereby increase the efficiency of hospital resources. The funds collected can also be used to improve hospital infrastructure including repairs of minor civil works, water tanks, electricity generator and incinerator, and to alleviate shortages of disposable items medicines and surgical equipment. In some places the revenue from user fees is used to install intercom systems and airconditioners in operation theaters and pathology departments, repairs of electric fittings and ambulances and preparation of information boards. Such funds are also used to contract out cleaning services to external agencies.

Three broad categories of user charges have been defined: the first consists of registration, bed charges, transportation and meal charges; the second category comprises charges for various diagnostic services; the third category specifies rates for different medical procedures and surgeries. Accommodation is typically graded into different categories, such as OPD/general ward, paying ward and private ward in an ascending order of service level. The rate structure for a given service varies according to the type of ward occupied by the patient. People possessing certification that identifies them as belonging to income groups falling below the poverty line are exempted from paying for health services in public facilities and entitled to get treated in the general ward only. However, as discussed later, the implementation of this rule has been the most serious area of neglect in the administration of the entire user fee structure. Some other special categories of people like government employees, freedom fighters, patients of medico-legal cases are also exempted from fees and this list varies in each state. The people belonging to such categories are exempted subject to furnishing of appropriate documents. Sometimes it is on the discretion of the medical officer of the concerned hospital that such exemptions are made.

Despite the similarity in the framework of user fee administration, there are interesting variations across states in the practical implementation of the user fee system. Amongst the states covered, Uttar Pradesh and Orissa are implementing the user fee system in full force and the detailed case studies are presented subsequently. The other extreme is that user charges have not been introduced yet in Tamil Nadu and Gujarat. In Gujarat, in 2002, there was a notification to levy user fee but due to political pressures, the plan was abandoned. Implementation in West Bengal has been relaxed as a result of which almost every user has free access. When the user fee was introduced in Karnataka, there was tremendous agitation from the people against it, but in due course of time people have realized that the service quality has also improved. Nowadays people are getting used to the harsh reality of the prevailing situation and are willing to pay if the quality of services is better.

An assessment of the user fee was made in relation to several indicators. Differential fee structure was looked at in relation to equity in access to healthcare. Barring Karnataka where user charges are uniform in all the districts, charges in other states are different both district-wise as well as on the basis of paying capacity of the user. Outpatient department registration charges vary between Re. 1 and Rs. 8, highest being in Uttar Pradesh. In addition, in Uttar Pradesh registration charges are revised upwards at the rate of 10 per cent per annum with a minimum increase of Re. 1 annually. Bed and other charges also vary from state to state.

One issue is the control over revenues from user financing—whether it remains with the institution or is it shared with other institutions or state projects. It is important because if the fee revenue or a part of it is returned to the general treasury, this acts as a cost to the local community and a potential issue of opposition for user financing. We find that the control over collected funds varies. Hundred per cent control is retained by the collecting institutions in most of the states with the exception of Uttar Pradesh where only half is retained by the institution since the remainder is transferred to the state treasury. Thus Uttar Pradesh hospitals collect the highest amount through user fees but get to retain only a part of it.

On the issue of equity and access of services to the poor and vulnerable, the interviews reveal that there are a number of ways of identifying the poor but an administratively simple method of identifying poor patients is the BPL (below poverty line) card which is used for individual exemption. But in practice identifying the poor when they come for treatment is often based on the discretion of the attending health official. Therefore, not everyone in the free facility category is a BPL card-holder. Moreover, in a number of states only a percentage of poor have been issued BPL cards, the most glaring example being Uttar Pradesh. Discretion thus becomes operational in such a context to provide services to those who do not have the capacity to pay. The relatively poor seem to have automatically been excluded from approaching the public district hospitals mainly due to the entry barrier caused by the concept of the user fee itself without proper information sharing from the hospitals and relevant bureaucracy. There is no emphasis on informing the masses that these services are free for those who cannot afford it due to inadequate income or cash.

User charges were introduced in Orissa in 1997 as part of the health sector reform—which began in the mid-1990s—with a focus on 3 'm', i.e. maintenance, regularity in medicine supply and mobility. The objective of the introduction of user fee was to raise additional revenue for hospitals and grant more autonomy to the hospitals for operations and day-to-day maintenance. The user charges apply to all tertiary district-level government hospitals in the state. The Orissa case study covered the Capital Hospital of Bhubaneswar and Balasore District Hospital. Registered societies were set up for each hospital, which collect and retain the money for use within the hospital. The societies are given the flexibility to raise the existing rates or introduce fee for new services subject to the general guidelines. Guidelines are also applied on expenditure of the raised fund. The admissible areas of expense include repair and maintenance of civil works, purchase of essential furniture, purchase of medicine at the time of natural calamities and epidemics, hospital waste disposal and cleaning and maintenance of hospital.

The Madhya Pradesh case study covered a community health centre in the Sidhi district of Madhya Pradesh with 30 beds. User fee was introduced in the first referral unit in 1998 under the Rogi Kalyan Samiti. Rogi Kalyan Samiti is a local society like societies in other states, which monitors the system. In the past three years a total of Rs. 70,000 has been collected from user fee. Interviews and group discussions with the residents revealed that the hospital is being used for treatment of minor ailments and people are willing to pay amounts depending on their ability and current expenditure on private facilities. However, without a detailed household survey, it is difficult to conclude much from the interviews.

The West Bengal case study was conducted at the District Hospital, Barasat. The exit survey conducted with in-patients and out-patients in the hospital revealed that patients were willing to pay out-of-pocket to ensure better attention from doctors and staff and for availability of medicines. In West Bengal a patient gets exempted from payment if s/he can produce a certificate of lower income from an authorized person such as the Block Development Officer (BDO), local political leader, and so on. Influence of political environment was conspicuous in case of user fee collection. People coming with a certificate from a political leader are exempted from the fee. In this way many well-off people take advantage of this system. On the other hand poor and deserving people without access to such politicians are denied free health care facility.

The Rajasthan case study covered a community health centre in Sikar district with 30 beds. User fee was initiated in the FRUs in September 2001 under the Medicare Relief Society Scheme. Within three months, a sum of Rs. 30,000 was collected by way of user fee.

TABLE 7.1: USER FEE: A STATE-WISE COMPARISON

	Karnataka	*Orissa*		*Uttar Pradesh*	*West Bengal*	*Rajasthan*	*Madhya Pradesh*	*Gujarat*	*Tamil Nadu*
	Chikmanglur DH	*Balasore DH*	*Bhubaneswar SGH*	*Bareilly DH*	*Barasat DH*	*Ajigadh, Sikar Dst. CHC*	*Rampur, Sidhi Dist. CHC*	*Rajkot DH*	*Ambasamudam Taluka Hosp.*
User charges implemented	Since 1996	Since 1997	Since 1997	Since 2000	Since 2001	Since 2001	Since 1998	No	No
Facilities charged	Diag., special accom. Transport	Diag, special accom. Transport	Diag., special accom. Transport	Diag. Accom.	Diag. Trnprt.	Diag.	Diag, medical	NA	NA
Rate: Uniform or differential	Uniform	Differential district (wise)	Differential district (wise)	Differential district	Differential district	Differential district	Differential district	NA	NA
Average daily OPD (year)	NA	NA	816	530 ('01)	847 ('00-01)	NA	235	1813	840 ('00-01)
Average daily in-patient	230 ('00-01)	162 ('00)	101 ('01)	54 ('00-01)	97 ('00-01)	NA	20	302 ('00-01)	81 ('00-01)
Beds sanctioned	400	217	310	300	306	30	30	470	64

Bed occupancy ratio (%) (in-patient/beds sanctioned)	76	74	32	18	31	100% peak and 50% lean period	66	64	126
Registration fee (Rs.)	–	2	2	6	1	2	2	NA	NA
User fee collection (Rs.)	11,54,589 ('00-01)		33,13,168 ('00-01)	25,52,712 ('00-01)	9,60,000 ('00-01)	30,000 in three months	23,000 (Annual Avg.)	NA	NA
Hospital access to user fee revenue (%)	100	100	100	50	100	100	100	NA	NA

CASE STUDY 1: USER CHARGES IN BAREILLY DISTRICT HOSPITAL

The Maharana Pratap District Hospital and Dufferin Women's Hospital in Bareilly initiated user charges on hospital services, in its present form, in July 2000. A committee was constituted at the district level for the implementation of user charges comprising six to seven members. The chief medical superintendent presides over the committee, which includes the medical superintendent of the women's hospital, a representative of the chief medical officer, a representative of the district magistrate among others. Guidelines have been provided to the committee in accordance with which user fee may be charged and subsequently spent. The district hospital is given direct access to over 50 per cent of the revenues raised from user charges for improving service delivery subject to the approval of the committee and the remaining amount is deposited with the treasury. The district hospital can utilize up to 75 per cent of its share on various expenditure heads as per the norms, the balance 25 per cent is kept as reserve for contingency purposes.

Types of User Charges and Hospital Attendance

At present, all users are required to pay a registration fee of Rs. 6 with some exceptions such as holders of white card, medico-legal cases, ex-employees, and so on. Doctors and officers-in-charge are also authorized to exempt the poor—who cannot afford the charges—from payment. In-patients are required to pay an admission fee of Rs. 28 and bed charges of Rs. 6 per day in the general ward with an advance payment of Rs. 60. In the emergency ward, admission and three days of bed allotment is free. There are three kinds of wards—general, paying and private—with different levels of services. Rate structures of all service such as pathology and X-ray vary in accordance with the type of ward that the patient is occupying. Table 7.2 gives the various heads under which user charges have been collected in the year 2000-1 in the Maharana Pratap District Hospital, Bareilly.

Hospital officials admitted that the poor find it difficult to pay for the user charges but also argued that no one is denied

TABLE 7.2: RATE STRUCTURE OF USER CHARGES, IN MAHARANA PRATAP DISTRICT HOSPITAL

Service	*User charge in Rs.*		
	General ward	*Paying ward*	*Private ward*
Registration	6	6	6
Admission	28	28	28
Bed charges	6	28	105
Normal delivery	220	330	550
C-Section	330	550	880
Blood transfusion (Excluding blood charges)	55	–	110
Evacuations	220	–	–
Minor operation/biopsy	220	–	–
Drip induction	–	330	–

the use of hospital services as they are treated free of cost or according to their ability to pay. The senior officials and doctors exercise their discretion in exempting people from payment of user charges. Although people holding only a white card as certification of poverty are exempted from user charges, only a small percentage of the poor actually possess the card and an even smaller proportion is aware of the applicability of such rules in health services. Some may feel that an imbalance has been created in which the relatively better off population has gained access to better public health facilities and is therefore able to economize on expenses for private health services, which they had been incurring in the past. The poorer sections on the other hand, who had access only to free public health services earlier are now required to pay out of their pocket.

Average OPD attendance at the Maharana Pratap District Hospital (MPDH) was 390 patients per day and 140 patients per day at the Dufferin (Women's) Hospital (DH) in 2000-1. Out of a total of 1,70,087 out-patients at MPDH, 477 were treated free of cost in 1999-2000. In 2000-1, out of 1,41,852 out-patients, 449 were treated free of cost. Average number of in-patients in MPDH were 30 per day in 1999-2000, declining to 27 per day in 2000-1. Average number of in-patients at the DH were more or less the same—27 per day during 1999-2000 and 2000-1. The total number of beds were 300, giving an

TABLE 7.3: SOURCES OF COLLECTION OF USER FEE, MAHARANA PRATAP DISTRICT HOSPITAL

(*in Rs.*)

Month 2000-1	*OPD reg.*	*In-patient reg.*	*General ward*	*Pvt. ward*	*Paying ward*	*Operation fee*	*Pathology*	*Grand total*
Aug.	49,635	13,545	19,945	8,535	11,410	13,100	14,748	1,48,638
Sep.	69,610	51,795	30,705	7,230	10,005	18,675	15,436	2,63,516
Oct.	70,770	13,900	21,525	4,175	7,850	22,900	22,062	2,20,147
Nov.	52,940	50,765	24,515	4,950	4,375	14,850	7,975	1,83,355
Dec.	59,550	23,850	23,970	1,800	750	11,300	9,041	1,85,511
Jan.	50,050	12,700	17,240	8,925	5,425	17,050	6,508	1,57,958
Feb.	61,038	4,153	5,073	3,176	2,256	17,515	15,153	1,49,124
March	62,310	22,456	3,996	3,900	20,023	38,060	8,945	2,72,145
April	71,430	21,252	4,224	7,552	16,713	37,330	11,839	2,46,383
May	68,544	21,184	15,959	5,478	3,360	31,680	15,213	2,23,374
June	73,944	19,404	11,510	1,411	1,400	34,955	10,764	2,14,713
July	71,532	22,064	18,455	8,381	5,760	43,620	12,329	2,87,848
Total	7,61,353	2,77,068	1,97,117	65,513	89,327	3,01,035	1,50,013	25,52,712,

average of 9,000 bed days per month. Based on our estimates the average bed occupancy was 36,667 per month, resulting in a bed occupancy ratio of approximately 33 per cent per annum.[1]

Hospital users that were interviewed as part of the case study expressed a mixed view on user charges at the district level. Patients argued that for them government hospital is the only option for medical treatment and they would have to continue availing it, despite user charges, as they cannot afford anything else and at least they get some medicines free of cost. Some users, including a few in the general ward, admitted that they were willing to pay for ensuring careful attention from the doctors and other medical staff.

Utilization of Revenues Collected from User Charges

Hospital officials uniformly presented a positive view on the efficacy of user charges with some suggestions for improvement. According to them user charges have been very helpful in improving the operation and maintenance of the hospital. Direct access and control over resources has proved to be beneficial in improving the hospital infrastructure such as repairs of water tanks, electricity generator and incinerator, and to alleviate shortages of disposable items, medicines, and surgical equipment. The revenues collected have also been used to install an intercom system and airconditioners in the operation theatre and the pathology department, repairs of electric fittings and ambulances

TABLE 7.4: MAJOR EXPENDITURE CATEGORIES FOR USER CHARGES IN MAHARANA PRATAP DISTRICT HOSPITAL

(*in Rs.*)

Expenditure Head	*June 2001*	*April-June 2001*
Life saving equipment & electrical repairs	25,954	35,374
Civil works	2,00, 000	2,36,379
X-ray plate, chemicals, oxygen cylinder refill, etc.	1,382	2,764
Disposable items	35,757	1,29,807
Stationary & printing	16,099	16,099
Total	2,79,192	4,20,423

and preparation of information boards. Some of the funds have been used to contract out cleaning services to an external agency on an experimental basis. Table 7.4 lists the major categories on which revenues raised from user charges have been spent at the Maharana Pratap District Hospital in Bareilly.

The hospital however, has been unable to utilize all the funds that are at its disposal. In addition, officials expressed reservations about the stipulation as per which user charges can be increased at the rate of 10 per cent per year. Hospital staff too found this rule to be too rigid to implement, at least in case of OPD patients. The officials remarked that doctors are not proficient as managers and to an extent find it troublesome to manage revenues and expenditures with the help of the available staff.

CASE STUDY 2: USER CHARGES IN ORISSA

The health department introduced user charges in Orissa in 1997. It has been introduced in three categories of services, viz., diagnostics, special accommodation and transportation in the tertiary, district and district level hospitals. The districts were divided into three categories on the basis of their economic prosperity and slightly varying rates were fixed for the different categories. Registered societies were set up for each hospital and the user charges collected retained by the society for use in the hospital. People below the poverty line are exempted from payment. Similarly tests relating to the national programmes are not charged. The societies have been given the freedom to raise the existing rates or introduce rates for new activities. They also have the authority to utilize the funds, subject to general guidelines, viz., no spending on new construction, on major equipment or on hiring of personnel.

CAPITAL HOSPITAL, BHUBANESWAR

The Capital Hospital constituted a Society of Capital Hospital under Societies Registration Act 1960. The aim of the society is to facilitate, improve or streamline treatment, patient care, hospital services, training of personnel engaged in the health, repair and maintenance of assets of the hospital. The executive committee of the society fixed the user charges keeping in view the local demand and paying capacity of the local people. State Capital Hospital Society shared those rates with district-level hospitals. In the same way the district hospitals also established an independent registered society in each district. The earnings from user charges are supposed to be spent towards purchase of consumables and reagents, repair and maintenance and purchase of spare parts for existing equipment. The other admissible areas of expense are repair and maintenance of civil works, purchase of essential furniture, purchase of medicine at the time of natural calamities and epidemics, waste disposal and cleaning and maintenance of the hospital. Capital Hospital, has not employed any person for collecting user charges. The only cost involved is a monthly honorarium of Rs. 500 to the accountant for keeping records.

District HQ Hospital, Balasore

It is a 217 (199 free and 18 paying beds) bed hospital with nine wards. This hospital too introduced user charges in 1997. Capital Hospital initially fixed charges on different facilities at the Balasore District Hospital, but it has been provided with autonomy to change or modify the rates. There is a society called Zilla Swasthya Samiti under the chairmanship of the district collector of Balasore. The executive head of the society is the Chief District Medical Officer (CDMO) and its other members include the local minister and local NGOs. The Additional District Medical Officer (ADMO) as a member of the society decides on the patients to be exempted or charged. Normally those below the poverty line, emergency patients, medico-legal cases and retired government, employees are exampled from paying user change. Services for which fee is being charged includes use of ambulance, special cabins, X-ray, pathological tests, audiogram, ECG and OPD registration. Balasore District Hospital collects on an average Rs. 70-80 thousand per month. According to the CDMO, financial autonomy and ready money gives immense confidence to run the hospital. The hospital can now keep all equipment in working condition and all reagents and disposables can be made available.

Before the introduction of user fee, most equipment used to be out of order and the CDMO had no power to repair them. Therefore, service was uncertain to patients. Nowadays users are also satisfied and have gained confidence about the hospital. Capable users are paying much less compared to private places and are even ready to pay a more for better services.

The whole process of user fee collection, keeping accounts and expenditure is being monitored by Zilla Swasthya Samiti. The CDMO along with the ADMO decides the expenditure on developmental activities which is later passed by the executive body. The main expenditure heads are found to be POL and repair of ambulance; purchase of X-ray plates, lab chemicals, needles, ECG machine, stabilizer, washing machine and so on. This hospital does not spend any money on accounts of collection of user fees. It does not even pay any honorarium to the accountant who keeps records of all income and expenditure.

Balasore District Hospital is trying to give comfort to the patient by charging a nominal fee. Patients in the general ward can ask for a pedestal fan by paying Rs. 5 per day. The hospital is also introducing air-conditioned cabins.

Figure 7.1 theoretically confirms the impact of introduction of user fee on patient profile. The hypothesis based on practical

TABLE 7.5: NUMBER OF IN-PATIENTS FROM 1994 TO 2001, BALASORE DISTRICT HOSPITAL

	1994	*1995*	*1996*	*1997*	*1998*	*1999*	*2000*	*2001*
Jan.	5183	5520	5118	–	5576	4486	4614	5166
Feb.	4812	4772	4969	–	4766	4036	4457	4915
March	5376	4580	4932	–	5487	4358	5034	5456
April	5038	4779	4610	5134	5256	4280	5164	5165
May	5442	4642	5040	5643	5860	4538	5264	5361
June	5521	4965	5218	5189	5015	4516	4618	5150
July	5849	5715	5229	5502	5512	5319	4958	6072
Aug.	5994	5522	5151	5276	5696	5596	4974	5686
Sept.	5410	5132	5041	5346	5353	5805	4634	5624
Oct.	5185	5116	4808	5414	5335	5370	4688	5601
Nov.	5031	4754	5756	5799	5523	4857	4979	–
Dec.	4930	4947	5545	5448	6119	4570	5749	–

FIGURE 7.1: AVERAGE NUMBER OF IN-PATIENTS IN A MONTH (1994 TO 2001)

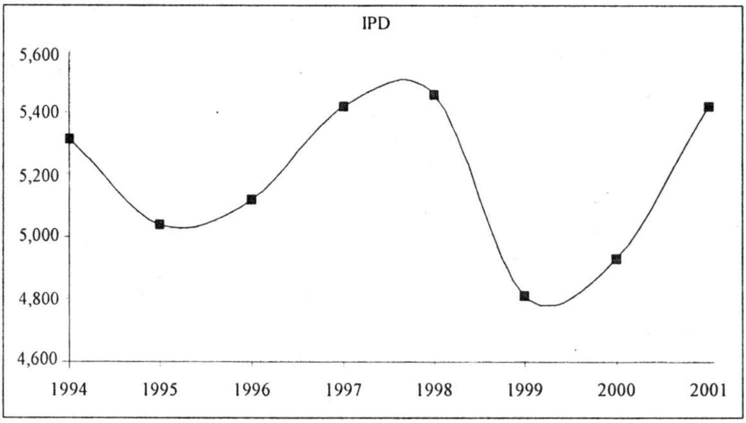

understanding is that in a public health care institution, patients' flow will decrease temporarily after the introduction of fee and will increase steadily after a time lag. This is because people can immediately see the burden of out-of-pocket expenditure and will try to find some other alternative. If the revenue collected is reinvested for the betterment of hospital services, then people find it useful and will come back with more confidence. User fee was introduced in 1997 and at the time the average number of patients was showing an upward curve. The upward movement started declining within a year of the introduction of user fee and this is the usual time lag taken for information to percolate down to the common people. Over the next one and half year it continued to decline further and reached a very low level. After that it started to rise again. This is because of the realization of the people that money collected through user fee is being utilized for the benefit of the patients and better facilities are now being offered. The pattern confirms the conclusion that we drew from exit surveys in this hospital. Patients reported that they are now getting better and timely services and therefore are more confident of being treated properly. They have also reported that medicine supplies have been regularized and there is rarely any difficulty in getting laboratory test done due to technical reasons.

CONCLUSION

The severe constraints of data availability combined with a survey of limited users makes it difficult to draw detailed conclusions from this case study of the user fee system. However, visits to the different hospitals, in-depth interviews with officials and users suggest that much more needs to be accomplished to increase the effectiveness and improve the equity implications of the user fee system. User fee administration and assessing exemption from user fee are poorly designed and implemented even more poorly.

While the financing of operations and maintenance through user charges has offered greater autonomy and flexibility to the health care institutions to improve the efficiency of hospital resources, visits to hospitals and interviews of officials reveal that not all possible gains are being exploited. Apart from political interference—sometimes on a day-to-day basis for purposes of winning political patronage—management and administration of user fee is an important concern amongst hospital officials. The existing staff is administering and managing the user fee system at present in the states surveyed. As the officials claim, medical doctors are not trained to manage resources and ensure their most efficient utilization. Also, user fee implementation is making increasing demands on hospital officials and staff to be more accountable and provide quality services to the public. Unless an overall improvement in service delivery is made in a short period of time, political opposition to user fee is likely to threaten the success of the system.

Another area of grave concern is the exclusion of the poorest and most vulnerable users from the public health care system. Interviews with users demonstrated lack of effective information dissemination to the users for maintaining accessibility by those who needed it the most. The user fee system exempts people below poverty line from all types of user fee. However, the poor are required to produce a white card, certifying their status to avail of free hospital services. Majority of the poor, however, do not possess the white card thus making the applicability of the rule almost impossible. Moreover, the few who do possess this certification are not aware of the rules regarding exemptions from user fee and seldom bring their cards to the hospital. In other words, a much more effective and reliable system needs to be developed for preventing the poor from exiting the public health care system than discretion based system currently effective in most hospitals. Lastly, it can be said that better conceptualization and implementation may lead to better results with improvement in services and thereby regaining of public confidence.

NOTE

1. This ratio does not take into consideration the number of in-patients treated free of cost.

APPENDIX 7.1

RATE OF USER CHARGES IN DISTRICT HOSPITAL, BALASORE

Lab Charges	*Rs.*
1. DC	8
2. TLC	8
3. Parasite	8
4. TRBC	8
5. HB	4
6. Platelet count	8
7. ESR	8
8. TB	4
9. CT	4
10. Stool (R & M)	8
11. Stool Ocult Blood	8
12. Urine (R & M)	8
13. Urine Special Test	8
14. Biochemical Blood Sugar	15
15. Blood Urea	15
16. Serum Bilirubin	15
17. Perferial Smear Study	8
18. CSF Exa	40
19. Skin Smear for AFB	15
20. Skin Scraping for Fungus	15
21. Seminal Fluid Analysis	10
22. Urethral Smear Pus-smear for Grams Stain	15
23. USG	100
24. X-Ray Section fee	
25. X-Ray 15″ × 12″	40
26. X-Ray 12″ × 12″	30
27. X-Ray 12″ × 10″	25
28. X-Ray 12″ × 8″	15
29. X-Ray $8\frac{1}{2}'' \times 6\frac{1}{2}''$	15
30. Dental Film 70 M	8
31. ECG	40
32. VDRL Blood	15
33. Indoor Admission fees	2

APPENDIX 7.2

RATE OF USER CHARGES IN CAPITAL HOSPITAL, BHUBANESWAR

Pathology Department	*Rs.*
1. Blood FBS	20
2. Blood PPBS	20
3. Blood PGBS	20
4. Blood RBS	20
5. Blood Urea	20
6. Blood Creatinine	30
7. Blood Cholesterol	20
8. Blood Bilirubin	50
9. Blood SGOT	30
10. Blood SGPT	30
11. Blood Alkaline Phosphate	30
12. Blood Total Prutin	30
13. Blood Albumine	20
14. Blood AG Ratio	20
15. Blood Uric Acid	40
16. Blood Triglyceride	50
17. Blood Blood HDL	50
18. Blood Lipid Profile	200
19. Blood Hb%	10
20. Blood ESR	10
21. Blood TRBC	10
22. Blood TWBC	10
23. Blood Platelet Count	10
24. Blood BT	5
25. Blood CT	5
26. Blood Sickling	10
27. Blood DC	10
28. Blood MF	10
29. Blood Comment on Peripheral Smear Reticulocyte Smear	10
30. Clot Retraction	10
31. Stool	10
32. Urine	10

33. Urine Pregnancy Test	30
34. CSF	50
35. Gramstain	20
36. Ascitic Fluid	50
37. VDRL	30
38. WIDAL	40
39. Toxo plasma	75
40. ASO	50
41. Rh. Factor	50
42. Mx. Test	20
43. Skin Fungus	20
44. FNAC	30
45. Seminal Fluids	20
46. Culture & Sensitivity	50
47. ECG	50
48. Computerized Stress Test (TMT)	350
49. 12″ × 15″ (Film Size) EACH	50
50. 12″ × 12″ (Film Size) EACH	40
51. 10″ × 12″ (Film Size) EACH	30
52. 8″ × 10″ (Film Size) EACH	20
53. Dental X-Ray	15
54. Upper GI Endoscopy	200
55. Abdominal Ultra	100
56. Filling of Tooth (Temporary)	30
57. Filling of Tooth (Permanent)	50
58. Scaling (Each Sitting)	50

CHAPTER 8

Public Hospital Reforms in Madhya Pradesh: Perceptions and Trends

GIRISH KUMAR

INTRODUCTION

The institutional structure developed for reforming public hospitals in Madhya Pradesh is known as the Rogi Kalyan Samiti (RKS), loosely translated as Patients Welfare Society. The RKS seeks partnership of all the concerned actors at the local level to raise funds for the upkeep of the public hospitals and, in turn, ensures their participation in the management of health services. The initiatives taken under the rubric of RKS comprise the introduction of user fee, contracting out of ancillary services, self-certification of poor and commercial use of the hospital land. It has also created space for the community-centered actions within the aegis of the new management structure. This paper is based on empirical evidence collected from 10 hospitals (case study method) located at different levels in five selected districts of Madhya Pradesh. Apart from taking stock of on-going health sector reforms in the state, the paper critically examines the decision-making process as well as sharing of responsibilities by different stakeholders under the aegis of RKS. It also aims at assessing the strength of institutional arrangements developed for ensuring transparency and accountability of the new management structure, and above all, its reach and impact in terms of catering to the health care needs of the primary stakeholders, more specifically of the poor patients and their level of satisfaction.

I

THE CONCEPTUAL FRAME, METHODOLOGY AND SAMPLING

A study of a new system for managing the government hospitals and health centres involves a close scrutiny of a complex system at work. It encompasses a large number of variables. This includes the rationale and extent of partnership, stakes of the key players involved, willingness of the state to allow the utilization of public institution and its infrastructure under the new management system, acceptance of the new set of rules by the users and above all, their (users) willingness to pay for the services available under the changed set-up. It can even be tempting to assess the effectiveness of the new system by making a comparative analysis 'of the costs and effects of clinical and public health' under both the previous and present institutional management practices but 'availability of such highly intensive data is rather difficult'[1] (Sankar and Kathuria, 2004). The paucity of relevant empirical data, i.e. the effective performance of the new system could, however, be overcome with the field observations and interviews of the patients, their attendants and local people of the town concerned. Besides, anybody who is a little familiar with the (mal)functioning of government hospitals and dispensaries in economically and socially backward states of the country can easily understand the import of the new system, even without visiting the hospitals where such changes have occurred.

Situated against this conceptual frame and context, the basic objective of this study is to document an innovative reform package involving public hospitals and present it before a wider audience. Apart from taking stock of the ongoing reforms in select hospitals in Madhya Pradesh, the paper seeks to critically examine the decision-making process as well as sharing of responsibilities by different stakeholders under the aegis of RKS. It also aims at assessing the strength of institutional arrangements developed for ensuring transparency and accountability of the new management structure. And above all, its reach and impact in terms of catering to the health care needs of the primary stakeholders, more specifically of the patients in general and poor in particular and their level of satisfaction.

The study is based on the data collected from ten hospitals (case study method) located at different levels in five selected districts of Madhya Pradesh. The sampling was purposive[2] and hospitals were selected following discussions with the concerned officials, including the director, health services, and a senior officer belonging to the elite central administrative services (of MP cadre) who happens to be the progenitor of this reform package. All the ten hospitals were visited during the six months beginning from September 2003. At each hospital, apart from interviewing doctors, including the chief medical officer, support staff, patients and their attendants, discussions were also held with the local elected representatives as well as government officials. Informal talks with common people and key informants in most of the district towns helped clear many doubts. The relevant facts and figures, for instance details of earning and expenditure of the RKS resources, were collected from these hospitals.

The paper is organized into six sections. The first section, as given above, provides the backdrop, context and the rationale of 'partnership' as well as its varying models evolved so far and put to work in different states of the country. The second section elucidates the conceptual framework of the study, its methodology and sampling as well as structural design of the paper. A brief political overview of the state of Madhya Pradesh highlighting its recent reform-oriented initiatives is presented in the third section. This section also gives a brief profile of the district/ study areas covered in the study. The process of unfolding of the new system under the aegis of the RKS in two hospitals under entirely different circumstances is documented in the fourth section. The major findings of the study, based on a comparative assessment of the functioning of ten selected hospitals are discussed in the fifth section. Put simply, this section aims at assessing the impact of the partnership on the functioning of government hospitals by highlighting the relative strengths and weaknesses of the new management system at work. The conclusions drawn are given in the last section.

II

A PROFILE OF THE STATE

In the wake of the reorganization of Indian provinces in the late 1950s, the state of Madhya Pradesh[3] was created in 1956. Spread over 4.43 lakh (1 million = 10 lakh) sq. km. and covering about 14 per cent of the country's geographical area, this centrally located province was the biggest[4] in a continental size country like India. And naturally, far more heterogeneous (Purohit, 1976) as compared to any other state in India. Nearly two-fifth of the area of the state was under forest cover and then it had the largest proportion of Scheduled Tribes, comprising 26 per cent (as against 7 per cent national average) of the total population. Until the early 1990s, the state had hardly witnessed any organized or protest movement, even lacked a distinct cultural and political identity. In terms of all development indices, it had always been clubbed with the BIMARU[5] states. It is still largely rural, dependent on subsistence agricultural farming with very low level of farm productivity. Land reforms were never on its agenda. Cooperatives and other village-level institutions such as panchayats (a three-tier institution of rural governance) never gained roots in its political soil. Green Revolution bypassed it; it did not witness the mobilization and consequent political empowerment of backward castes either. Neither could it create a sound industrial base for itself, despite huge mineral deposits. No wonder, it has the largest number of poor (people below poverty line in official parlance): 42.52 in 1993-4 as against the national average 35.97 (Planning Commission, 2002); it held

TABLE 8.1: HEALTH INDICATORS (VARYING YEARS)

	LEB	*IMR*	*MMR*	*BAHP*
MP	55.1	131	498	30.1
India	60.7	77	407	43.3

Source: National Family Health Survey (1998-9) and Ministry of Health and Family Welfare, GOI (Annual Report, 2000-01).

Legend: LEB: Life Expectancy at Birth (1992-6); IMR: Infant Mortality Rate (1991); MMR: Maternal Mortality Rate (1998); BAHP: Birth Attended by Health Professionals (1998-9).

30th rank among all 35 states and union territories. Madhya Pradesh was and is essentially a feudal state which has retained its feudal moorings in many ways.

Given its rigid social frame, relative backward political consciousness enforced with widespread poverty and deprivation, it is hardly surprising that it also faltered on the track of democratic decentralization during its two earlier phases in the early 1960s and in the mid-1980s (Kumar, 2002). It was also one of those nine states which remained highly (politically) unstable during 1967-71, witnessing as many as seven chief ministers and a brief interlude of President's Rule. Indeed, no other chief minister, except Digvijay Singh could rule over the state for two consecutive terms (10 years), a rare feat indeed and that too for an upper caste politician.

Digvijay Singh understood that such a deeply entrenched feudal society could not be changed unless external force was applied. In order to achieve the goal, a number of steps were taken. This included: creating multiple institutions/opportunity structures at the local level; putting programmes on their agenda with freedom to innovate at the local level; ensuring smooth flow of funds directly to them with the provision of combining resources and expertise of multiple stakeholders; and ultimately catalyzing social mobilization (Kumar, 2006). A series of innovative initiatives, including rural livelihood programmes, delivery of services and women's empowerment in particular, were introduced during Digvijay Singh's tenure. Well acknowledged by the UNDP, some of these programmes including the RKS received international (Global Development Network) awards too (*Hindu*, 26 December 2002).

STUDY AREAS

The 10 selected hospitals were taken from five districts, namely, Bhopal, Dewas, Khandwa (East Nimar), Indore and Ujjain. Of these, Dewas, Indore and Ujjain are contiguous; rather Dewas is equidistant from both Indore and Ujjain city. All the five cities have more than one million population, the biggest, however, is Indore (see Table 8.2) which also happens to be the commercial capital of the state. Bhopal, the capital city is well endowed

TABLE 8.2: PROFILE OF THE STUDY AREA

Districts	*Area (in 000 sq. km.)*	*Total Population*	*Sex Ratio*	*Population Density*	*% Literacy*	*% Urban Pop.*
Ujjain	6,085	17,09,885	940	281	71.18	38.74
Dewas	7,025	13,06,617	932	186	61.04	27.35
Indore	3,899	25,85,321	911	663	74.82	71.57
East Nimar	10,743	17,08,170	936	159	61.71	26.95
Bhopal	2,770	18,36,784	896	663	75.08	80.53
MP			920	196	64.08	26.67

Source: Census of India, 2001.

with several management and technical institutions, including a medical college and a prestigious cultural centre. It is also known for its commercial activities besides having a sprawling industrial township (having 1.5 lakh people) of one of the public sector undertakings. Altogether, it has ten big public hospitals[6] and as many as 36 big, medium and small size nursing homes and hospitals, including a trauma centre, an eye and a heart hospital.

Dewas is a district town, located at a distance of 160 km. from the state capital. It has a fairly large tribal population. It used to be a sleepy, non-descript town endowed with perhaps a solitary sign-post of development—a federal government organization for printing (Indian) currency notes. Lately, during the last decade, it has emerged as a new industrial hub. The number of hospitals and nursing homes are modest (see Table 8.3) as compared to big cities like Indore or Ujjain. The latter is one of the ancient cities, a religious place dotted with several temples; it has an ancient observatory too. With a fairly large Scheduled Caste population, Ujjain parliamentary seat is reserved for this community.

The city of Indore, as mentioned above, is the biggest in our sample. It has more than five dozen hospitals, including 21 Ayurvedic, Unani and Homeopathic hospitals. Among all the three neighbouring district towns/cities, there is one thing in common: the presence of Jains, a community of merchants essentially, who control the commerce and trade in all these three cities, though numerically they are small, comprising not more than 3-4 per cent of total population. Their trading practices may not be different than those of other business communities,

TABLE 8.3: DISTRICT-WISE NUMBER OF ALLOPATHIC INSTITUTIONS AND BEDS (1998-9)

Districts	*Distt. Hospital*		*Urban CH*		*CHC*		*PHC*		*Total*	
	No.	*Beds*	*No.*	*Beds*	*No.*	*Beds*	*No.*	*Beds*	*No.*	*Beds*
Bhopal	1	210	2	125	2	30	10	12	15	377
Dewas	1	270	2	30	2	60	25	55	30	415
Indore	1	100	4	242	3	96	26	48	34	486
Khandwa	1	290	1	111	7	210	46	46	55	657
Ujjain	1	57	5	161	2	60	20	34	28	826
MP	42	9,148	74	3,609	342	10,338	1,690	2,069	2,305	27,347

Source: www.mp.nic.in/des/scmp2000/scmpT113.htm

but they are well-known for their philanthropic activities. The same is true of Badnagar,[7] a tahsil-level small town located at a distance of 50 km. from Ujjain city. Several charitable educational and health institutions are run by this community in Indore city which is also known for the publication of a fairly influential and widely read Hindi newspaper (*Nai Duniya*).

Khandwa, the headquarters of East Nimar, is situated in south-western part of the state in the range of Satpura Hills. In fact Khandwa is the only railway station which falls on all the northern, southern, eastern and western routes. Put simply, it has direct rail links with all the four metropolises in the country. Yet devoid of any major industrial activity, the district is known for its subsistence agriculture. The landholdings of the majority of peasants are small and agricultural labourers are in sizeable number. Among its pride of places is the Lady Butler Hospital,[8] one of the oldest in the region. A PHC at Pandhana tahsil, located at a distance of 20 km. from Khandwa was also covered in this study.

III

THE RKS: GENESIS AND EVOLUTION

The decision to form the RKS was, however, a bureaucratic intervention made amidst the scare of plague looming large over the western part of Madhya Pradesh following its outbreak in Surat, a major commercial city in neighbouring Gujarat, in

1994. Then, the Maharaja Yashwant Rao (popularly known as MY) Hospital, the 750-bed district hospital of Indore was in throes of an unprecedented crisis. It was infested with thousands of rats, carriers of the plague virus. The fear of plague had necessitated a thorough clean-up operation involving a major task—trapping the rats and killing them. The district treasury did not have the money for this operation. Frustrated with the lack of resources, the then district collector of Indore decided to make use of an obscure official directive, permitting the collector to set up RKS. Put simply, it meant involving people[9] in running the hospital as also for the welfare of patients. The RKS was formed; an appeal was made to people and charitable organizations for donating money for the purpose. The response was quick and soon the money started flowing. Within a month Rs. 48 lakh (Rs. 4.8 million) was collected. That was enough not only to tide over the immediate crisis but also to refurbish the old hospital and put it under a different management system. The district administration, doctors, nurses, para-medicos, donors, people's elected representatives and the press—all the possible local-level actors decided to join hands together to keep the momentum on for the upkeep of the hospital and improve upon its existing services. And thus, RKS was given a formal shape and authority.

Highly impressed with this novel programme, Chief Minister Digvijay Singh issued a directive for the implementation of this programme in all district-level public hospitals in the state. The RKS was reportedly formed in 'more than half of the nearly 1,200 public hospitals in the state' and 'an estimated Rs. 37-40 crore' (1 crore = 10 million) was 'raised across undivided Madhya Pradesh in the five years and spent on the improvement of the hospital' (*India Today*, 8 January 2001). Under the new management system, the patients are charged user fee for the health care services they avail of. However, the poor patients, those who cannot afford to pay this fee are exempted and treated free of cost. To cap it all, they do not have to bring any testimony to support their poor state of being; their self-certification is taken as a valid proof of their poverty. The chief minister described these innovative steps—charging user fee and self-certification by the poor—as two new concepts in health governance and also claimed their wider acceptability by the people and the new management (ibid.). The success of RKS triggered further innovative steps such as allowing commercial use of hospital land.

The 'system works', observed a UNICEF team which assessed the impact of RKS towards the end of 2000. The system, however, is not without lacunae. For, it was pointed out that 'overall control of the local RKS bodies remain in the hands of the collector and if he is not interested in health care then the whole thing might just drift'[10] (ibid.).

In contrast to Indore, the RKS at Badnagar tahsil (a sub-division, an administrative unit below the district) hospital began on a different note. Interestingly, it all started with what is described as a clear mis-match between the training of personnel and the jobs they handle. Trained basically as a surgeon, Dr. L.A. Kapadia, the medical officer-in-charge of Badnagar Hospital was at pains when he found himself posted in this hospital which did not have even a sanctioned post for a resident surgeon. That was Badnagar Hospital in 1979. Dr Kapadia began his innings as a physician. Obviously, he was unhappy for not getting an opportunity to put his surgical skills to use. Although there was nothing to prevent him from practising surgery, the biggest handicap was the unavailability of basic infrastructural facilities. A decade after, a few young Jain businessmen of the area approached him. Fired with philanthropic zeal, these young men sought his advice on what to do with the money they were eager to spare themselves, and also willing to mobilize from the business community settled over there. Having been involved in occasional charitable work, they formed an organization in 1990 called Sahyog Yuva Sangathan (SYS) to channelize their philanthropic urge. It was registered in 1991 but by then SYS had already generated enough resources to donate an operation table and a suction pump—two essential components of a surgeon's workplace. Earlier they used to provide nutritive food supplements to the poor patients.[11]

As mentioned above, its seedlings had been planted much before the Indore initiative,[12] and accordingly, it has moved on a different track. Earlier, the partnership was forged (for the welfare of patients) unofficially and without any organizational frame. Therefore, the RKS at Badnagar could take proper shape only after the official pronouncement to this effect. On 1 June 1996, almost two years after the success of the Indore experiment, the state government instructed to form RKS at the 'tahsil' level. It was quickly acted upon at Badnagar. On 30 June 1996, it was formed with the sub-divisional magistrate as its executive director, the local MLA as ex-officio chairman and Dr. Kapadia as its secretary. Among the other notable members were the presidents of the local *janpad* panchayat (intermediate level of three tiered decentralized institution) and the municipality respectively. Four months later the RKS Badnagar was officially registered.

A fund was set up to monitor the amount thus collected. Private donations were allowed to be put in the same fund. The fund for all practical purposes was operated by the secretary who is also vested with the cheque signing authority. The secretary in turn is accountable to the executive committee of the society to which he reports in its monthly meetings, chaired by the SDM. The GB meets once in three months (quarterly) and the local MLA chairs it. Prior to 1998, the Badnagar *janpad* panchayat president used to preside the general body meetings. It became operational on 1 January 1997.

The registration fee was fixed at Rs. 2 in case of OPD (a token consultation fee) and Rs. 5 in case of indoor patients who were admitted. Likewise for indoor patients, the bed charge was Rs. 5 per day, Rs. 30 for X-ray (of all types) and Rs. 150 for surgical operations. The user fee for the last item, i.e. surgical operation, was raised to Rs. 250 in February 2001. Similarly, there were varying charges for different types of laboratory/pathological tests. On this account alone the RKS earned Rs. 7.51 lakh[13] during the last seven years ending March 2002. This cannot be termed as profit since the cost of all the inputs, including expensive chemicals are borne by the RKS. At the same time, the RKS has ensured all the facilities under one roof. Prior to the formation of RKS, this was not possible since the treasury rules in the state, as in most of the states, did not permit the facility to retain the funds collected on account of user's charges.

With this amount, the hospital was renovated and essential medical equipment were procured. Next year a pathological block, X-ray block and two special wards were constructed from the area development fund of a local member of the state legislative assembly. The state health department also sanctioned 14 beds for male and 12 beds for female respectively to the hospital. Over and above, the RKS was also instrumental in getting a medicine shop constructed inside the hospital campus. By auctioning it, the RKS raised Rs. 7.21 lakh. At the same time it ensured the availability of essential drugs in the campus and that too round the clock. Similarly, by auctioning a canteen inside the hospital campus RKS received Rs. 3.32 lakh.

Associated Facilities

In April 1997 a 'Sulabh Complex' was constructed[14] to extend bathroom facility to patients and their attendants. Subsequently, under the auspices of the Annapurna Seva Samiti,[15] a mess facility was also launched for the patients and their attendants. This shows the evolving characteristic of RKS. Everything was not planned in the beginning. On the contrary, it started on a modest scale to provide relief to poor patients. Gradually, it went on expanding, adding necessary structures as per the felt need of the patients.

IV

THE RKS AT WORK: TRENDS AND PERCEPTIONS

Earlier the public hospitals were plagued by many problems: for instance, posts lying vacant for long; inadequate supply of essential materials such as X-ray films or essential chemicals to run pathological laboratories, etc. Still they had everything required to run a modicum of curative services: staff, infrastructure, annual budget, supply of medicines and other sundry materials from the government depots. Undoubtedly, there were shortcomings in every sphere. But a feeling of demoralization had gripped the doctors in general, more particularly at the level of chief medical officers (CMO). 'There was a crisis of confidence', to quote a relatively young doctor serving at the Bhopal-based JP Hospital. 'It was really embarrassing when as the CMO, I would not be in a position to sort out even sundry/

mundane grievances that would cost not even Rs. 20. It is not a big amount. But can a CMO go on spending, howsoever little amount it is, practically every day from his own pocket? It was a helpless situation. For everything you had to report to the Directorate of Health Services and wait endlessly for their response. Meanwhile not only would the patient suffer but the staff would be sitting idle.[16] For they would not have the wherewithal to attend to their work', commented a CMO of one of the sample hospitals while elaborating the manifestations of the crisis.

Decentralization of Authority and Responsibility Sharing

Now the doctors do not have to wait. They have sufficient funds at their disposal. They do not have to take prior permission for petty expenses. In fact, in some hospitals (JP for instance) enlightened CMOs have decentralized the system of responsibility sharing and decision making as well. Accordingly, all the departmental heads have petty cash to take care of their day-to-day expenses, including minor repair works or for buying, for instance, a bulb or tube (for lighting). They can decide what else their priorities are and if it does not involve substantial expenditure, they can go ahead. They need not rush to the CMO. Likewise, the CMO is also authorized to spend within a prescribed limit without seeking prior approval of the district collectors and chairman of the RKS executive committee at the district hospitals. 'It is this sense of empowerment which in turn has helped me instill discipline among the support staff and doctors alike. All the services have been streamlined. Everybody has some work to do. And I do not have to run after them. Of course, I go on my rounds, twice a day which in a way helps build pressure on those who still are lagging behind', the same CMO explained.

Decentralization has worked as the functioning of departments has improved, commented the dean of MGM Medical College, Indore. The MY Hospital is an associate hospital of this medical college. To a large extent, it has helped to overcome day-to-day hassles.[17] Regretably, this assertion of the dean was not shared by others. In fact, discussions with a few departmental heads and medical superintendents of other associate hospitals in the sprawling campus of this medical college revealed that they were hardly consulted by the former. 'They do not have voice in the RKS of MY Hospital. There is a lack of integrated approach; the Dean focuses on his own (orthopaedics) department', rued a retired MS of one of the hospitals. A visit to the orthopaedics department confirmed this allegation. The cleanliness, number of equipment, general upkeep—this department wore a different look as compared to any other department of MY Hospital. The lack of team spirit in the functioning of the present dean was pointed out by other doctors, too. 'Lack of promotional avenues for doctors including middle level supervisory staff as well as complete absence of a mechanism for reward and punishment (read incentives for best performing doctors and staff and in reverse case disciplinary, if not punitive, action against the erring or negligent staff, including doctors) has added to the maladies of the hospital's functioning', to quote a group of doctors at Khandwa.[18] In continuation, they also dismissed the notion of decentralization at work in their hospital. Paradoxically, the 'team spirit' was noticeable among the doctors but they seemed alienated from the RKS-driven reforms. Rather, a few of them were contemptuous of it, calling the RKS a big hoax. Lack of team spirit was also noticeable at another Bhopal-based hospital, at Ujjain and Badnagar too, though the last in the row has earned kudos for taking several other RKS-linked successful initiatives.

Expenditure and Earning Patterns of RKS

On an average, there is 5-10 per cent increase in the annual income of the hospital, thanks to the RKS-induced collection of user fee. A look at the balance sheet of the district hospital, Khandwa reveals that its overall earning has gradually gone up. For instance, during 1995-6, its total earning from all sources[19] was Rs. 1,16,452 but by 2002-3, it registered five times growth, notching a figure of Rs. 6,15,007. This is true of practically all hospitals observed. Clearly, there was willingness on the part of the patients to pay for the services they were availing.[20] And decidedly, the service delivery mechanism must have improved otherwise people would not have paid. The pattern was by and large the same in practically all the selected hospitals.

What use were they making of these additional resources, collected in the form of service charges? Again at the Khandwa hospital, it was paltry Rs. 30,341 in 1995-6; Rs. 1,33,588 next year and Rs. 5,16,918 in 2002-3 on half a dozen heads, including miscellaneous expenses.[21] Incidentally, the last item, i.e. miscellaneous expenses, seem to be heavy, followed by medicine purchase and the cost of repair and construction. There are, of course, variations in income and expenditure pattern across the hospitals studied. For instance, the inventory of expenditure procured from Ujjain district hospital is too big to compare with Khandwa. At Ujjain, the balance sheet shows heavy expenses on account of staff salary, their travelling and conveyance allowances as well as remuneration allowances, totaling a little over Rs. 5.62 lakh in 2001-2. Similarly in the same period, the expenditure on three items—building maintenance, sanitary material and repair and maintenance—totalling Rs. 10 lakh was spent from the RKS fund. Incidentally, there has been recurring expense on building repair and maintenance, year after year starting from 1997. Although they did not give satisfactory explanation[22] to this end, but went on happily pointing out to the fact that earnings have gone up and accordingly the expenses, but the latter never exceeded the former. To illustrate this point, it should be noted that in the financial year 1996-7 the total income from various sources was Rs. 14 lakh whereas the corresponding expenditure figure was about its half. On the other hand in Dewas, the expenses incurred during 2000-1 was equal precisely to its earning, at least according to audit report. The audit report also shows that of the total of nearly Rs. 2 million spent on various items, a little less than Rs. 3 lakh were found spent on civil work (repair and maintenance of the building and hospital premises), painting, furniture and electrical appliances. Incidentally, just a year after (i.e. during 2002-3), again on these four items alone, over Rs. 12 lakh (of the total Rs. 32.22 lakh) was spent. It is also not clear as to what stands for 'contingency' on which a huge amount (Rs. 8.23 lakh) was found incurred during the same financial year.

However, a retired superintendent of MY Hospital expressed serious concern over the misuse or wanton use of resources[23] by the current dean. Several such instances were brought to our notice, attesting to the fact that to the 'felt needs' are underlined by the man at the helm of affairs. And this was not a problem specific to MY Hospital alone. Expenditure on unnecessary items, or wrong priorities fixed by influential doctors (read head of the institution or their hangers on), or simple wasteful expenditures—these were noticed in most of the hospitals. That the head of the institution might go wrong in the exercise of his/her authority does not seem to be of concern in any management structure. This is true of RKS too. For, the new management structure either lacks a check and balance provision in-built in the system or it has been rendered useless. In either case, it is regrettable.

Barring a few exceptions, the fee or donations collected are not being properly utilized in most of the hospitals covered in the study. It all depends upon the perception of head of the institution. Although it is not a discovery *per se*, it belies the conception that if there are additional sources of income and the management is broad based, including representatives of practically all stakeholders, the situation would dramatically improve.

Patient Satisfaction

The public hospitals are flush with resources, thanks to the willingness of patients to share the cost of treatment by paying service charges, that is user fee. They are paying for the simple reason that services are available now. In the pre-reform period, a visit to the hospital meant free consultation only. And only the poor would seek admittance or avail a modicum of IPD facilities.[24] Earlier, in any case, patients had to buy all the essential items required for surgical operations.[25] Over 400 patients and their attendants across all the sampled hospitals were interviewed and a great majority of them expressed satisfaction with the functioning of the hospitals. Narrated variously, the substance of their response was that the quality of services had gone up and several facilities had been added; the doctors and nurses were also found to be more attentive. This was however not true of the patients at Ujjain and MY Hospital, Indore. Paradoxically, the MY Hospital which witnessed the birth of the RKS was in a bad shape. In fact, it was passing through a series of crises, one after another, so much so that even the then medical superintendent voiced his unhappiness with the state of affairs, pointing fingers on the lower-level staff. 'Despite too much insubordination, one can take no action either against junior doctors or support staff, more particularly sweepers', he added. The lower level staff on the other hand blamed the administration for the privatization of services. It was indeed chaotic. It may also be mentioned that the affairs of the MY Hospital had already received a lot of negative media coverage (charges of corruption included) therefore the hospital administration had instructed its staff to not to speak to outsiders on hospital affairs. The superintendent and the dean spoke of 'political interference' too. This point was also raised at a few more hospitals, including at Badnagar and JP Hospital where RKS-driven reforms have paid great dividends.

Transparency and Accountability

The dissatisfaction among the lower and middle level staff, including junior doctors was to a large extent, a function of their negative perception of the RKS. The RKS was formed following a government fiat without taking hospital staff in general into confidence. They were neither directly involved in the day-to-day decision-making of RKS nor did they gain opportunity to attend RKS meetings. Thus, remaining devoid of any insights into the nature of changes that began surfacing, they were suspicious, even mistrustful for this otherwise innovative step. Privatization of certain services, appointment of a few staff and collection of user fee further confused them. Indeed, some of them began fearing retrenchment. Although none of the permanent staff have lost their jobs, nor was it the stated objective of the RKS, their collective fear has not completely been allayed. On the other hand, they have not been able to comprehend the objectives or the goal of the RKS. Above all, the lack of transparency (regarding purchase of equipment or contracts awarded to private parties) and accountability on the part of the new management structure towards the hospital staff has reinforced their suspicion. The tall claims of introducing changes in the overall management of hospital ring hollow to their ears when they find the doctors, as usual, attaching more priority to their private practice than spending the required numbers of hours in attending patients in the wards or in the OPD section.

Is it any wonder that the hospital staff, in general, seem to be alienated from what is going on under the auspices of the RKS? Noble exceptions apart, in most of the sample hospitals the lower and even middle level staff seem to be completely oblivious of the objectives of the ongoing reforms in their respective workplaces. If the degree of mistrust or dislike, as we noticed, was greatest among the staff of MY Hospital, followed by Ujjain, the alienation was also noticeable in the response and attitude of the staff even in those hospitals like Badnagar, Bhopal or Khandwa, where RKS-induced changes are more conspicuous. Over and above, the peculiar mind-set of the pampered government employees at the lower level particularly causes conflicts and tensions. As the superintendent of the MY Hospital pointed out: they do not realize that the additional staff (sweeper for instance) is hired for the better upkeep of the hospital, therefore instead of cooperating with them, they either abdicate their responsibilities, passing the buck or creating mischief. In either case, the regular hospital employees keep the RKS-recruited staff at arm's length.

LEADERSHIP AND CHANGE

The effectiveness of the new management structure to a large extent depends upon the perception and vision of the head of the institution. In the given context, it is all the more complicated since the chief medical officer of the traditional health administrative set-up also assumes the responsibility of the secretary of the RKS. This brings the leadership question to the fore.

Undoubtedly, the leadership attributes vary from one person to another, depending on the context and the functional nature of the organization. For the purpose of this study, these qualities have been quantified with reference to the following points: Have they succeeded in transforming 'I' into 'We', combining self-interest and common good and striking a balance between immediate and long-term goals? Do they listen to their subordinates and are open to criticisms and suggestions? What is the extent of authority and responsibility sharing? Are they making judicious use of the resources generated through the user fee?

If the performance of the sample hospitals is measured on a ten-point scale in the light of the specific questions raised above, supplemented with the general observations, JP Hospital with 8 points would score the first position, quickly followed by Badnagar Sadar Hospital. At the bottom of the list would be the Ujjain, MY Hospital and Katju Hospital, scoring 2-3 points. The grading for the rest would be average in the range of 4-5 points. Among them, however, Dewas and Khandwa hospitals, I found to be slightly better despite the absence of a dynamic leadership but both these hospitals have committed staff, particularly lab technicians and nurses as well as a couple of doctors.

CONCLUSION

The RKS heralded a major initiative to reform the near-defunct government hospitals in Madhya Pradesh. As a result, new structures have been created, additional resources mobilized, and more facilities have been assured to patients and additional hands are available to serve them without adding to the financial burden of the state. Steps have been taken to enforce accountability of the staff, including doctors, as also transparency in the use of available resources, though on both these counts there is much to be desired of. Above all, the patients appear to be by and large satisfied, though we came across a large number of unsatisfied patients too, and for obvious reasons, at Ujjain and MY Hospital, Indore. The monitoring is limited as it is more attuned to observing procedures rather than regarding it as an exercise in ushering dynamism in the functioning of the RKS. The proceedings of the RKS executive committee meetings would testify to this fact. Indeed, the main actors of the RKS, noble souls apart, seem to be complacent, happy, satisfied, even saturated with their performance, as if they have reached the end of the journey; there is nothing beyond. This does not mean that the reforms have failed to motivate staff, fired by the zeal and sense of duty. They are there and so are the leaders: disciplinarian, visionary, trustworthy who inspire confidence among the team members. But they are in very thin minority. Thus there is hardly any organized effort to bring about change in the behavioural pattern and work ethics; inject the sense of duty and mould the traditional mindset of the health functionaries in order to make them the *de facto* agents of change. Admittedly, the task is far from being completed. Yet, the fact remains that less than a decade is too short a period to internalize the essence of the reform by all the stakeholders. The signs however are disturbing. For instance, instead of making RKS a truly broad-based body vested with decision-making powers, its scope has been reduced. For instance, RKS is focused on the management of locally used resources (user fee, donations); it has no role in the hospital administration powered by the annual budget received from the state government.

Notwithstanding such shortcomings, the RKS has been able to change the mindset of the people that the state is a doer and service provider and also that these services could be availed of without paying or sharing the cost. At the same time, it has in-built safety net for poor patients too, though it is largely discretionary in nature. Most importantly, the RKS has demonstrated that instead of allowing the huge health infrastructure created in 1970s and 1980s to go waste in the face of ever-shrinking budgetary allocations, these institutions could be given a new lease of life by changing the rigid official rules and regulations. The bottom line is that if we create space for community-centred action, encourage experiments and engage people in meaningful participation, varying patterns of health governance will emerge. To cap it all, follow-up actions must be ensured since one-time intervention will fail to yield desired results.

NOTES

1. This is due to a number of reasons including the conceptual problem, the use of different determinants—whether to 'use the monetary expenditure on health' only or consider also 'non-health-system determinants such as income and education levels' as well as the extent of public hygiene or even access to safe drinking water and nutrition level. For an excellent reading on the issue, see Murray and Frank (1999); Savas (2000) is equally useful but he has discussed 'partnership' in the context of privatization alone.
2. For the simple reason that like all reform-oriented processes, the progress is slow and tardy too in case of translating the ideals of RKS into practices. After discussions with the concerned officials and other knowledgeable sources, the impression I had gained was that practically in all the district-level hospitals something or other had been added to their physical infrastructure (new equipment, renovation of old buildings, etc.), thanks to the additional resources now available under RKS, but its underlying assumptions in letter and spirit are yet to be internalized in most of the hospitals. Therefore, it was decided to select any ten from a dozen or so hospitals identified as those where visible changes had occurred. Then, restricting the sample size to 10 was also a logical outcome of time and budgetary constraints.
3. The geographical boundaries of this state have undergone changes many times. In 1956, it was created by merging the areas falling under two states, namely, the Central Provinces (CP) and Vindhya Pradesh. Altogether, the new state had five distinct regions, and prior to independence, some of its constituent units were governed under the provisions of the British India acts while the rest were under the control of hereditary rulers (princely states) and were essentially politically backward. In fact, the level of political and economic development, including their exposure to the functioning of local-level institutions in the various units of the state were at variance among its constituent units.
4. In 2001, it was divided into two states. By carving out predominantly tribal areas, spread over 16 districts in eastern and south-eastern part of Madhya Pradesh, a new state called Chhattisgarh was created. The state still has a substantial tribal population.
5. Loosely translated as 'perpetually sick', the term BIMARU is used both as an abbreviation and also as a connotation in Hindi. Literally it refers to an individual or an organization which is unable to compete with the healthy ones owing to its continued sickness. As an abbreviation, it stands for Bihar, Madhya Pradesh, Rajasthan and Uttar Pradesh. Together they represent the Hindi heartland of the country

and in terms of all possible social and economic development indicators, they stand far below relatively developed states in the southern and western part of the country. Due to their continued backwardness, they are referred to as perpetually sick states.

6. Included among these are six special hospitals: two Unani and Ayurvedic hospitals, one for TB patients, yet another exclusively for women (Sultania Lady Hospital), one for the victims of the Bhopal gas disaster of 1983 (Bhopal Memorial Hospital and Research Centre), and another associate hospital of the Bhopal Medical College (Hamidia Hospital). Besides these there are four hospitals in the general category. Of these, two, viz., JP Hospital and Katju Hospital, were studied.
7. It should be noted that the total population of Badnagar town, the headquarters of the tahsil having the same name, is approximately 35,000. Being numerically large and having big stake in the land and the state politics, the Brahmins and Rajputs dominate the area. Together, they constitute about 25-30 per cent of the total population. The Jains, the business/trading community, comprise about 3-4 per cent of the total.
8. Named after the wife of the then British governor, the Lady Butler Hospital is relevant for us in more than one way. In first place, it is the product of a classic instance of PPP. Secondly, it is a major sign-post of RKS-sponsored success. This hospital was established way back in 1929, largely with the initiative of Sir Arthur Butler, the then British governor of Central Provinces and Berar. Having moved by the plight of women, dying in large number during childbirth due to lack of hospitals, he decided to set up one. For the stated purpose, however, he urged the local notables to contribute resources to which he added government grants—all mentioned on a plaque at the entrance of the hospital (see also *East Nimar District Gazetteer*, 1969).

   This old hospital later became the gynaecology department of the Khandwa District Hospital. It was lying almost defunct for almost fifteen years when the reform package started unfolding. Thanks to the resources raised through RKS, this hospital was thoroughly renovated and its past glory was restored.
9. It was a massive exercise by all means. In order to kill the rats and clean the premises, it was decided to close the hospital for over a month. It necessitated, in the first place, evacuation and shifting of hundreds of patients to several hospitals, both in the government and private sector, which was swiftly done. All the exit routes were sealed and then poisonous gas was used to kill the thousands of rats. There were tonnes of garbage in the hospital including old, rusted and broken furniture and beds—all rejected and discarded items which were lying there for years. It took 40 trucks to remove the garbage from the compound, the then district collector revealed in a personal interview

(20 September 2003 at Bhopal). Subsequently, the hospital was refurbished. Its earlier layout was chaotic; for instance, the mortuary was next to the drug store. Therefore, as per the requirement and convenience of the patients and staff everything was relocated. The MY Hospital got a new look and new lease of life.

10. Anybody who is a little familiar with the institution of the district collector would testify to this fact. As the fountainhead of the district administration, the collector directly or indirectly controls most of the district-level bodies. But it is nearly impossible for a collector to pay special attention to a particular committee on a regular basis. Yet if a collector has concern for the health sector, s/he is in a position to mobilize funds and reduce dependency on the government. At any rate, the rider remains, that is, if the collector is interested and on his agenda health remains a high priority programme. The reverse is equally true. That once the progenitor is gone, the programme, howsoever innovative, might collapse sooner or later. In any case, the very dependence on an individual is an antithesis to the process of institutionalization.
11. Personal interview with some of the office-bearers of SYS as well as Dr. Kapadia during my first visit to Badnagar in January 2002.
12. Raising some additional resources from the donors and users was not something novel that had occurred at Badnagar or MY Hospital alone. In bits and pieces, it had earlier been attempted elsewhere too. A nominal user fee (Re. 1 for OPD and Rs. 5 for IPD) was introduced at the Chacha Nehru Children Hospital, Indore, way back in 1985 with the due approval of the then chief minister (personal interview with Dr. B.C. Chapparwal, a former medical superintendent of the hospital at Indore, 27 September 2003). In 1992-3 under a 'Child Survival and Safe Motherhood Programme' (sponsored by the Global Task Force in which the UNICEF was also involved) staff members of Dhar (adjacent to Indore district) hospital had collected funds to set up a dignified Women and Child Department (WCD) as a part of the hospital. At that time, from the collected funds, even the Dhar Hospital was given a facelift. Even WCD, to some extent, was operating like RKS. What was the motivational factor? I asked. 'They were expecting incentives and appreciation too from the sponsoring agency', a key official of the Department of Health, Bhopal explained (personal interview, Bhopal, 10 September 2003).
13. The average number of patients handled by the RKS Badnagar is over 100 per day. In 1996, the total number of patients was 41,039. Among them 34,822 had come to OPD (that is, those who came for consultation only); 4,537 were admitted, including 1,230 cases of child delivery. The total number of patients went up to 42,291 in 1998 but last year it came down to 41,224. Thus from the registration

fee alone the hospital gets, on an average, Rs. 1 lakh annually. Considering the annual budget of this hospital, which is said to be approximately Rs. 30 lakh, it is nothing. Of this, it should be noted, not even 2 per cent is provided for the patient's care. The reason is not budgetary constraint alone, which is very much there as in other states but in case of Badnagar there is some thing more, that is, the number of available beds maintained on account of RKS is more than double than the sanctioned strength of 26 beds. Patients flock in large number, such is the fame of the hospital and more notably, the name of its legendary surgeon, that the hospital had to install more beds. The occupancy rate of beds is cent per cent. It is here, inside the wards that the quality of patients' care and standard of (medical) treatment are put to real test. The ambience of the hospital becomes crucial in case of post-operative care. For, half of the IPD cases (i.e. those who are admitted in different wards, but excluding maternity ward) handled by the hospital is surgical in nature. In 1996, 1,680 surgical cases were handled of which 1,319 were major cases. The number of such cases has gone up since then. In 2001, for the sake of record, it was altogether 2070, including 1,722 major surgery cases.

14. Drainage facility was also provided, though this facility was not up to the mark owing to some fault in laying the slopes. Notwithstanding this fault, the local unit of the Public Works Department played a notable role in the designing and construction of this complex.
15. 'Annapurna Seva Samiti' is perhaps the latest addition to the hospital campus. This too has an interesting background. It is well known that people (patients and their attendants) mostly coming from the villages either happen to be poor or men of modest means. In either case, they cannot afford the food available in roadside eateries. Consequently, they are forced to cook their meal on earthen *chullahs* (ovens). This not only creates unhygienic conditions but also adds to the environment pollution (imagine the black smoke and leftover littered around the hospital campus). To overcome this problem, again a few enthusiastic philanthropists raised money and a mess was set up in August 2000, three and half years after the RKS became operational at Badnagar. Annapurna is managed by a retired schoolteacher with the help of five full-time employees, including cooks and cashier. Practically, everyday a vegetarian meal for 50-60 people is cooked which is provided at a token rate of Rs. 5 per person. The charge is fixed, not on the basis of per plate rather as much as any one can eat. The food was tasty and sumptuous. We ate our lunch the day we visited (it was an unannounced visit). In any case, there were plenty of people to testify to both the quality and quantity of the food served at Annapurna.

People have donated money and continue to do so. To provide food to the needy is considered to be a noble, pious act in Oriental societies. Driven by this feeling, individuals sponsor either lunch/dinner or both a day by paying Rs. 750 (in case of lunch alone it is Rs. 500 and Rs. 350 for dinner only) on special occasions, such as birthday of their children or on their wedding anniversary. Then, there are individual donors. For instance, a prosperous farmer from a nearby village, who stayed in one of the wards for a couple of days after an operation, was so impressed, we were informed by the manager, that he donated 25 quintals of wheat to Annapurna. The manager is a retired person and therefore has time at his disposal. He spends nearly whole day in supervising the catering services. He also owns a shop close to the entrance of the hospital, which is otherwise run by his assistant. Besides, there are always one or two volunteers around to give him a helping hand. The monthly budget of Annapurna is Rs.15-16 thousand but it earns only around Rs. 10 thousand out of the 'token' charge of Rs. 5 per meal. The deficit is covered by donations. 'We want to make it self-sufficient', the manager told us, 'by putting enough fixed deposit in the bank. Annapurna already has Rs. 2 lakh as fixed deposit in its name. We will raise contributions to reach a level where the interest accrued from the fixed deposit would be enough to take care of its running expenses.' It needs mentioning that though Annapurna is very much a part of RKS, on a day-to-day basis, it operates under the control and supervision of its manager who reports to the executive committee monthly meetings of RKS. 'Providing subsidized food to patients and attendants', the official guidelines for RKS reads, also happens to be one of the stated objectives of the RKS, therefore, the mess facility has come up practically everywhere, as an associated accessory of the RKS. But nowhere else did we find the mess facility equal to what we observed at Badnagar. In fact, it was worst at Ujjain (see, *Times of India*, Mumbai edition, 28 January 2004) and to a lesser degree at Indore. It was the same as the rest of the hospitals excluding Dewas where the mess facility was slightly better, covered in this study.

16. 'Earlier, the X-ray films allocated to the hospital would be exhausted in three-four months. Then in the rest of eight-nine months, I would be sitting idle. In the absence of X-ray films, I would not have any work to do. The patients would suffer and I would feel bad. I would have resigned had there been better working conditions in the private sector at my level. Besides, the fear of losing a government job with residential accommodation always loomed large in my mind while stepping out of the hospital. Above all, I was getting my salary regularly. Yet, honestly speaking, it was a real pain. Quite often I felt sick. Now, my hands are full round the year, thanks to the RKS. And,

patients are equally happy,' a radiologist posted in one of the hospitals in the capital city told us about the dramatic effect RKS had on his life and work in a government hospital.

17. Initially, the head of departments at MY Hospital were given Rs. 1,000 as contingency amount; it was subsequently raised to Rs. 2,000 and finally, Rs. 5,000. They are also authorized to call tender and buy equipment essential for their respective departments without prior permission, of course within a prescribed limit. This has instilled a sense of trust among colleagues (personal interview with the CMO, MY Hospital, Indore, 25 September 2003).
18. The doctors serving at Khandwa Sadar Hospital have set up a 'tea club' where they meet every evening. Not only does the club offer them an opportunity to enjoy a little break over a cup of tea, it also serves as a forum for free exchange of opinion and information sharing among the doctors who regularly discuss administrative, professional as well as personal problems. Most importantly, this forum is also open to the local private practitioners. Over the years, the club has matured as an institution, promoting trust and fraternal relations among its members. The acting CMO was kind enough to permit me to use the occasion to have a group discussion with the doctors available on 25 January 2004, the day I visited the hospital. The impression I gained from the discussions with them was that the RKS had simply touched upon just one of the maladies, that is, lack of resources. But it has failed to address other equally important problems.
19. This means earning from the following services: donations, OPD, IPD (admission fee from those who were admitted in the hospital), private ward, operation theatre/labour (child delivery), X-ray, pathological laboratory, ECG, ICCU, blood bank, etc. By and large, the heads were the same in the case of other hospitals, though some had a few more sources such as rents from shops constructed in the campus, ambulance services, parking lot/cycle stands, sale of tender forms and bedding contract, interest on savings, and if there were some more technical services available like sonography (in Ujjain).
20. According to Mushtaq Ali, on an average, Rs. 2-2.5 lakh are collected monthly at the JP Hospital (Bhopal) as user fee alone. The daily collection is deposited in the local branch of the State Bank of India after 12 p.m. Ali was appointed on an ad hoc basis in 1999 to take care of day-to-day accounts, correspondence, computerize the details of RKS-related activities; also prepare agenda of executive and general body meetings of RKS, and later write minutes of these meetings.
21. The six expenditure heads were stationary, machinery, medicine, repair and construction, return of fare (collected earlier in excess, hence returned in two financial years) and a broad miscellaneous expenditure.

22. The working environment at this hospital was different largely because of an enthusiastic medical superintendent. When I first visited the Ujjain district hospital in January 2002, the RKS of this hospital was earning nearly Rs. 2.50 lakh per month from user fee alone. The charges were almost in the same order as in Badnagar. With the user fee and donations raised under the auspices of the RKS, the hospital had added a burn unit, costing Rs. 7.80 lakh. It had enhanced the services rendered by X-ray and pathological units. And people were gladly paying since charges were almost three to four times lower than the prevailing market rates. 'For an electrocardiogram one has to pay just Rs. 15 while the private nursing homes charge Rs. 50-60 for the same. For blood sugar test in the hospital it is Rs. 8, the corresponding market rate is Rs. 30. With these facilities assured in the hospital, thanks to RKS, the business of private nursing homes has gone down,' the medical superintendent said to underline the comparative advantage of the RKS at Ujjain. It should be noted there are about two dozen nursing homes in Ujjain city, including half a dozen big ones with each having 50 beds. We also learnt that the local chemist association has donated medicines worth thousands of rupees. Similarly, a big textile industry donated 100 blankets worth over Rs. 70 thousand. To cap it all, recently, the governing body of the RKS sanctioned 8 air-conditioners for the hospital in just three days. 'It would have taken several months to get the sanction from the health department,' a beaming medical superintendent told us and added, 'getting as many as 8 air-conditioners sanctioned at a stretch from the government department was simply unthinkable' (Personal interview, 8 January 2002).
23. For instance, an intensive surgical care unit worth little over Rs. 3 million was constructed and was lying unused for eight months since its operational details were not worked out. At the same time, the diagnostic lab was privatized on the plea that an auto analyser (for testing blood samples on a large scale at a time) would cost Rs. 1 million. To the present dispensation, either it was a useless investment or there was lack of resources. At any rate, it was a wrong assessment. The lab has an important place in medical education since the students acquire hands-on practice but this fact was simply ignored, without caring for the future of medical students.
24. The budgetary provisions for the patients' care was half a rupee per out-patient per day (that is, the patients who come for consultation only) and two and half rupees for in-patients (those who are admitted and occupy beds) and add to it a rupee more in case of bigger hospitals. 'These rates were fixed up almost a quarter of a century ago and were never revised,' the CMO of Ujjain hospital told us (January 2002).

25. This includes even items like gloves, catgut (surgical sutures), naso-gastric tube, catheter, even cleaning material like liquid iodine. Some of these items are quite expensive. For instance, a small bottle containing 100 ml of liquid iodine costs Rs. 40. Now the attendants of patients do not have to run from a chemist's shop to another since every thing is provided by the RKS. And since purchasing is done in bulk, the relative cost of these materials goes down and quality is ensured. People gladly pay this amount for the very simple reason that it is nominal as compared to operation fee charged by nursing homes. Besides, those who cannot afford it, they are treated free of cost. At least, half a dozen poor patients testified to this fact (interview with Dr. Kapadia and scores of patients at Badnagar, during visits in 2002 and 2004).

REFERENCES

Baru, Rama V., *Private Health Care in India: Social Characteristics and Trends*, New Delhi: Sage, 1998.

Bhat, Ramesh, 'Issues in Health: Public-Private Partnership', *Economic and Political Weekly* (henceforth *EPW*), 30 December 2000, pp. 4706-16.

———, 'The Structure and Utilisation of Health Services: An Inter-State Analysis', in Mohan Rao, ed., *Disinvesting in Health: The World Bank's Prescriptions for Health*, 1999, pp. 129-44.

Duggal, R., S. Nandraj and A. Vadir, 'Health Expenditure Across States—Part I', *EPW*, 15 April 1995, pp. 834-44.

Kumar, Girish, 'Constitutionalising Panchayats: The Response of State Legislatures', Occasional Paper No. 4, Centre de Sciences Humaines, New Delhi, 2002.

———, 'Promoting Public-Private Partnership in Health Services', *EPW*, 19 July 2003, pp. 3041-5.

———, *Local Democracy in India: Interpreting Decentralisation*, New Delhi: Sage, 2006.

Krishnan, T.N., 'Access to Health and the Burden of Treatment in India: An Inter-state Comparison', in Mohan Rao, ed., pp. 212-30.

Misra, Rajiv et al., *India Health Report*, New Delhi: OUP, 2003.

Nandraj, S. et al., *Private Health Sectors in India: Review and Annotated Bibliography*, Mumbai: CEHAT, 2001.

Planning Commission, *National Human Development Report*, New Delhi: OUP, 2002.

Purohit, B.R. 'Madhya Pradesh: Politics of Princely Alliances', in Iqbal Narain, ed., *State Politics in India*, Meerut: Meenakshi Prakashan, 1976.

Qadeer, Imrana 'The World Development Report 1993: The Brave New World of Primary Health Care', in Mahan Rao, ed., *Disinvesting in Health: The World Bank's Prescriptions for Health*, New Delhi: Sage, 1999, pp. 49-64.

Rao, Mohan, ed., *Disinvesting in Health: The World Bank's Prescriptions for Health*, New Delhi: Sage, 1999.

Sankar, Deepa and Vanish Kathuria, 'Health System Performance in Rural India: Efficiency Estimates Across States', *EPW*, 27 March 2004, pp. 1427-33.

Savas, E.S., *Privatization and Public-Private Partnerships*, Delhi: East West Press.

Shrivastava, P.N., *Madhya Pradesh District Gazetteers, East Nimar*, Government of Madhya Pradesh, Bhopal, 1969.

World Bank, *World Development Report*, New Delhi: OUP, 1993.

CHAPTER 9

Making of a Primary Health Centre: The SEWA Rural's Experiment of NGO-GO Partnership

PANKAJ SHAH, LATA DESAI AND SHOBHA SHAH

INTRODUCTION AND BACKGROUND

SEWA Rural (SR), started in 1980, is a voluntary development organization based upon the ideals and ideas of Swami Vivekananda and Gandhiji. It endeavours to reach out to and assist the 'poorest of poor' through various health and development programmes based on community needs and available manpower. The activities in rural, tribal areas of South Gujarat were initiated by a group of young professionals that had education and experience both in India and abroad.

The focus of all programmes have been vulnerable members of society such as the poor. More specifically, the focus has been on vulnerable members of families such as women, children, and the elderly. The different activities include health, vocational training, education, women's development, and so on. SR also seeks to ensure that values are preserved and self-development, in a broader sense, is achieved for staff and employees involved in SR work.

An attempt is made to incorporate and balance the three basic principles of social service, scientific approach, and spiritual outlook into all of the organization's activities.

THE AREA

SR works in a predominantly tribal area. The adult population is largely marginal farmers and landless labourers with more than one-third living below the poverty line. The male literacy rate was as low as 30 per cent while the female literacy was around 20 per cent in 1980. The morbidity and mortality rates were very high since basic health services were practically non-accessible to most of the rural people. Basic concepts related to health and hygiene awareness were also significantly lacking. Preventable diseases like anaemia, infection, and tuberculosis caused a large number of deaths among infants and women. The infant mortality rate (IMR) was 172 while the maternal mortality ratio was more than 700 per 1,00,000 live births. The mortality rate was much higher among women in all age groups than of that among men. Almost 68 per cent of women died by the age of 45 as compared to 52 per cent among men.

Beginning with a Hospital

SEWA Rural initiated its activities in October 1980 by starting a 30-bed hospital generously given by a Jhagadia-based local organization, Kasturba Medical Aid Society. Even though overall rural development was the ultimate objective, hospital activity was the first step as the founding group members had expertise in the medical field.

Launching of the Community Health Project

Once rapport and credibility were established within the community, the medical work extended beyond the hospital walls. On 2 October 1982, a Community Health Project (CHP) was initiated in ten villages covering a population of around 11,000. The programme was built around a mobile dispensary, which had a team of nurses, doctors, and a compounder. The mobile provided curative health services. The focus was on tuberculosis (TB) follow-up and maternal and child care.

TAKING CHARGE OF JHAGADIA PHC AND PHASES OF GOVERNMENT COLLABORATION

This was an unprecedented example of collaboration between an NGO and GO where a voluntary organization was given the responsibility of running a PHC with 100 per cent grant-in-aid.

The process of collaboration gradually evolved in three phases (Annexure 9.1). The SR team members put in conscious and deliberate efforts during these different phases to ensure that the nature of responsibility, monitoring mechanisms, reporting systems, and funding arrangements between SR and the government were clearly defined and passed in various government resolutions.

The salient features and factors, which were found to be crucial in the successful collaboration in these three phases, have been detailed out as below.

First Phase (1982-4)

In 1982, SR, through a liaison with the state government, got the technical and administrative control of the entire village-level health functionaries. These functionaries included the *anganwadi* workers (AWW), *dais*, and community health volunteers (CHV) of ten selected villages around Jhagadia covering a population of about 11,000.

Second Phase (1984-9)

In 1984, SR received a Government of India (GOI)/United States Agency for International Development (USAID) fund for five years to address both curative and primary health care covering 39 villages in the Jhagadia Block. These 39 villages are referred to as project villages. The population coverage gradually increased from about 21,000 people in 1984 to 40,000 in 1986. With the responsibility of providing total health care as per the PHC set up, SR was required to undertake all the national government health programmes and meet all of their designated targets.

One AWW, one to two *dais*, and one community health volunteer were designated for every village with a population of about 1,000. For a cluster of 4-5 villages (sub-centre), a team of one male and one female health worker was appointed to provide all outreach services, which included ante-natal care (ANC), post-natal care (PNC), immunization, growth monitoring and supplementary nutrition of young children under ICDS, family planning (FP), health education, control of communicable diseases like malaria and tuberculosis, and treatment of minor ailments. A cadre of supervisors supported them in the field while Central support was provided through the PHC headquarters and the SR hospital in Jhagadia.

> DRIVING FORCE
>
> - Minimize duplication of services and resources
> - Develop a model PHC that can be replicated
> - Bring policy changes in management of government PHCs which can effectively address the needs of the poor
> - Bring changes through practice rather than just advocacy

SR professionals believed that by adopting a government PHC, along with its working structure and targets, it would provide opportunity to bring changes from within. It was thought that such an experience would go a long way in bringing about policy-level changes to develop effective government PHCs. SR also believed that since it was already working in the area of primary health care, adopting a PHC would help to minimize duplication of services and confusion among the workers and the community.

THIRD PHASE (1989-99)

In 1989, after completing five years of providing total health care services to 39 villages (population of 40,000), the government granted SR's request to take total responsibility of a formal PHC in Jhagadia. The salient features of the resolution have been highlighted in Annexure 9.2. This entails complete management of the PHC as per the norms of the government.

The government, however, allowed some flexibility in bringing out innovations with subsequent changes in the government's basic structure and system. For instance, SR negotiated for some autonomy in order to set its own targets. This led to the integration of the PHC and *anganwadi* staff, revision of management information systems, and reprioritization of programmes. The government resolutions and agreement clearly laid out powers, roles, and responsibilities of different stakeholders.

FOURTH PHASE (1999 ONWARDS)

In 1999, SR entered a new phase of collaboration with the government and the United Nation's International Children Emergency Fund (UNICEF), where it planned to set up a First Referral Unit (FRU) covering the entire Jhagadia block (population of 1,60,000) under the Safe Motherhood Programmes. Again, the emphasis was to develop a model FRU to upscale the lessons learned at the district and state levels. SR is currently interacting with the six PHCs and the entire health machinery of Jhagadia taluka by motivating and supporting them to innovate, particularly in the area of safe motherhood and newborn care at the community level.

INTERNAL PREPAREDNESS

The decision of collaborating with the government in 1984 and taking over a PHC in 1989 happened over many internal debates and dialogues raising serious concerns and apprehensions. The concerns were as listed below:

- Collaborating with the government in a formal way will affect the autonomy of the institution, and the programmes would be subservient to government rules and orders. It was felt that government intervention might affect the principle of serving the poorest.
- Government collaboration would bring 'government culture' and would affect the spirit of volunteerism.
- There was concern about the relationship with the community. SR views the community as an active partner in the programmes and encourages people to contribute time and money.
- There was apprehension pertaining to the character and outlook of the service providers, i.e. staff. Many feared that exposure to government working style, salary, formal training, and interaction with government staff might affect the overall mentality of SR staff, which SR has so carefully nurtured and developed.
- There was concern as to how the NGO fraternity would

view SR. Would SR be branded as siding with the government?

These concerns were not easy to resolve. The SR staff was engaged in debates to understand the overall objective of reaching the poorest of the poor and to develop mechanisms to preserve the organization's values and culture. Thus, the staff's overall commitment to identify issues and to work on them it on a continued basis created an internal environment of consensus, spirit and mandate to go forward for the collaboration with the government. One of the core group member's experience working with the government and SR's long-term association with positive minded government officers facilitated the process.

The Process of Taking Over

To make the collaboration meaningful, effective, and satisfactory, several steps were taken. The first one was to understand the basics of the government system and procedures. SR spent considerable time in understanding PHC functioning, including its system of reporting, supervision, programme monitoring, and financial monitoring. A senior medical officer and co-ordinator stayed for two days in one of the better government PHCs of the district in the early 1980s. They tried to learn the details of its daily working. SR provided additional time and energy for orienting its staff and developing a collective vision of working with the government.

COMMUNITY-BASED HEALTH PROGRAMMES: INNOVATIONS, COVERAGE AND IMPACT

Within five years and eleven years ahead of schedule, SR had reached the government's 'Health for All by 2000' goal. By the end of the first phase of five years (1989), utilization of services had reached the desired goal of 'Health for All by 2000' (HFA). In-service data (as seen in Annexure 9.3) indicates that quality and coverage of service utilization reached high levels, and the impact on most mortality rates had been considerable. For example, IMR was reduced from 172 to 42. Birth rates also fell significantly (from 35 to 21) with an increased effective couple protection rate (from 35 to 69 per cent). Most of the communicable diseases and epidemics were fairly controlled. Prevalence of severe malnutrition among children was also substantially reduced (from 16 to 2.5 per cent). There was a higher level of awareness about various aspects of basic health in the community, as seen from the increase in coverage of maternal care (from <25 to >85 per cent) and immunization coverage (from <10 to >95 per cent).

During the second phase of ten years, efforts were made to improve the quality of services and to increase health awareness among families and the community. Emphasis was placed on the importance of having good health, measures to preserve health, early identification of risk factors, and referral of complicated cases to the hospital where quality services are available.

MATERNAL AND NEWBORN CARE

Maternal and newborn services are considered together because, apart from being conceptually a continuum, even the provision of these services is difficult to separate. However, SR has introduced some modifications over the years and maternal and child health services have developed into a standardized package. Maternal care includes ante-natal care (ANC), care during delivery (intranatal care or INC), and care of the mother for 42 days after delivery-post-natal/postpartum care (PNC). Newborn care (NBC) is simultaneously provided to neonates up to one month.

Antenatal Care

The percentage of women covered satisfactorily for ANC check-ups (encompassing all the critical components: early registration, timely and complete ANC check ups and high risk referral, full course of iron and TT injection) increased from less than 25 per cent in 1982-3 to over 90 per cent in 1998-9. It has remained around 85 per cent for the last five years. Delivery preparation was found to be satisfactory for almost 80 per cent of the women.

THE CRITICAL COMPONENTS OF QUALITY ANTENATAL CARE ARE . . .

- Early registration -<12 weeks.
- Minimum 3 check-ups of pregnant mother within 24 weeks, 24-28 weeks, after 36 weeks.
- Regular monitoring of blood pressure and haemoglobin.
- Advice for proper nutrition and avoidance of tobacco and alcohol.
- Utilization of full course of iron folic acid tabs and TT injection at proper intervals.
- Identification and referral of high risk mothers.
- Preparation for delivery.

Intranatal Care

Preparation for home delivery by families is a critical component for safe motherhood and child survival. Having a trained birth attendant and timely identification and referral of high-risk mothers facilitates safe home deliveries.

CRITICAL COMPONENTS OF PREPARATION FOR HOME DELIVERY BY A FAMILY

- Expected date of delivery known.
- Procurement of pre-sterilized delivery pack.
- Packet of clean cloths made ready in advance.
- Trained *dai* of the village informed in advance.
- Readiness for referral if any complication develops at the last minute.
- Which hospital? (Where is a Caesarean facility available?)
- Which vehicle? (Availability of local transport).
- Arrangement for money (in advance).
- Who would accompany the woman?

SR has identified practising *dais* from all villages and provided intensive and practical training and retraining on techniques of safe delivery. SR developed a disposable home delivery pack in 1987 to facilitate the process of safe delivery. Following its successful experimentation by SEWA Rural, the Government of

Gujarat introduced this pack all over the state. Secondly, trained persons have been conducting more than 85 per cent of home deliveries safely for the past 15 years, whereas less than 20 per cent were trained in 1982-3. Moreover, the sterilized delivery pack is currently being used for conducting home deliveries in 90 per cent of cases. Hospital delivery increased from less than 10 per cent in 1984-5 to about 37 per cent in 1999-2000 with most of these hospital deliveries being complicated cases.

Postnatal Care

The postnatal follow-up is particularly done to look for post-partum bleeding and purpurial sepsis. In post-natal care, SR gives vitamin A supplement, especially to mothers already deficient due to pregnancy and delivery. The mother's health is followed up again after six weeks postpartum in order to ensure that she is physically and psychologically recovered and that she is able to give adequate care to the newborn. The coverage of postnatal visits within the first week of delivery is being maintained at around 90 per cent. During the lactation period and/or up to six months after delivery, mothers are also provided supplementary nutrition through the *anganwadi*.

Newborn Care

The importance and relevance of neonatal care is realized from the fact that 70 to 75 per cent of all infant deaths occur in the neonatal period. Two-thirds of these babies die during the first seven days due mainly to low birth weight and infection.

SR has developed a special package of newborn services, which can be managed at home. Every newborn child is monitored for seven consecutive days after birth and then on the 14th, 21st and 28th day with the help of *anganwadi* workers.

Due to these multiple interventions and special support provided for newborn care between 1998 and 2000, the infant mortality rate came down to 41 from 64, while there was a substantial reduction in neonatal mortality rate, which came down to 29 from 45.

CRITICAL COMPONENTS OF NEW BORN CARE

- Promotion of use of sterile delivery packs at birth.
- Drying and wrapping babies at birth.
- Exclusive breastfeeding from day 1.
- Birth weight on day 1.
- Checking of newborn for danger signs everyday for the first week and then every week for one month (total 10 visits).
- Education and awareness of family members for danger signs (feeding problems, infections, poor activity, etc.) by putting pictorial posters on the wall at home.
- Early identification and referral of critical babies to hospital.

CHILD HEALTH SERVICES

In 1984-5, SR, while collaborating with the government in providing comprehensive healthcare services (PHC responsibility), also took charge of the Integrated Child Development Scheme (ICDS) in its project villages.

A clear indicator of the effective and quality childcare services provided by the organization was indicated in the declining CMR from 12 (1982-3) to 3.8 (1999-2000). It could also be seen in the reduced IMR from 172 (1982-3) to 41 (1999-2000). Thanks to the emphasis on certain measures like immunization, oral rehydration solution (ORS), weaning, and prompt referral, there was an early decline in the post-neonatal mortality rate (PNMR) (from 52 in 1982-3 to 24 in 1993).

ICDS

The main thrust of the ICDS is the health and development of pre-school children and mothers. The major activities under this programme include providing supplementary nutrition to pre-school children and to pregnant and lactating mothers, pre-school education, health and nutrition education to mothers, growth monitoring, immunization, and treatment of minor ailments. These activities are carried out with the help of AWW at the village level. A helper also assists the AWW.

More than 95 per cent of the children in the eligible age group (under 6 years) are registered under the ICDS programme as per the in-service records. Vitamin A coverage (2,00,000 IU every six months) was maintained at about 95 per cent, which helped in reducing the incidence of vitamin A deficiency in the area.

The proportion of children that were malnourished was 16 per cent in 1982-3, and this came down to 11.5 per cent in 1988-9, 4.2 per cent in 1992-3, and then has remained at between 2 and 2.5 per cent from 1994 onwards.

IMMUNIZATION

Immunization is one of the key health components, particularly for maternal and child health. In 1982-3, the coverage for all primary vaccination was less than 10 per cent.

The 'Health For All by 2000' vaccination target was achieved in SR areas by 1989-90, which was a decade ahead of the government's targeted date. The coverage of all six primary vaccines reached almost 100 per cent from the baseline in 1982-3.

Among children ages 1-4 in-service data reflected that there were no deaths due to post-measles complications, no deaths due to tetanus or diphtheria, no cases of polio since 1986, and only sporadic cases of measles and whooping cough since 1990.

CURATIVE SERVICES

SR placed great importance on curative services, as it is one of the felt needs of the community. These services were provided at the village level as well as at SR's Kasturba Hospital.

Village Level: Initially (1982-4), curative services were initiated through the mobile dispensary on a weekly basis. Gradually, community health volunteers and paramedical workers took over this responsibility. The diseases treated at the village level were common illnesses like diarrhoea, dysentery, fever/malaria, common skin infections, common cough/colds, and minor injuries. In a population of about 40,000, about 40 village-level volunteers and paramedical workers treated around 25,000 to 30,000 patients each year.

Hospital Level: Kasturba Hospital provided valuable referral support. Over the years, people of the surrounding 1,500 villages utilized the 75-bed Kasturba Hospital. The hospital is equipped with facilities such as a laboratory, a blood bank, operation theatres, X-ray and sonography technology, an emergency and intensive care unit, a labour room, and a neonatal ICU. The services are provided largely in the areas of general medicine, tuberculosis, obstetric and gynaecology, paediatrics and ophthalmology through a team of medical specialists and paramedics. Presently, more than 65,000 outdoor patients are seen while more than 6,000 admissions take place each year. More than 800 deliveries are conducted, and about 6,000 surgeries are performed every year. More than 1,000 new patients are diagnosed to have TB, out of whom 70 per cent are based on sputum positivity. All of these services are largely subsidized or free to the needy.

Communicable Disease Control Programme

SR has been taking active measures in its project villages towards control of communicable diseases. Special focus has been given to malaria and tuberculosis control. SR has been able to make these programmes, began in 1984-5, effective through community education and awareness, community participation, and introduction of several innovations.

Malaria Control Programme: The malaria programme included meticulous collection of slides, provision of presumptive and radical treatment, bioengineering techniques to prevent water collection, distribution of fish seedlings, and ensuring timely treatment.

There was a 50 per cent reduction in the proportion of *P. falciparum* infection at the end of the project period. ABER also declined and has remained around 12, which indicates a satisfactory level of malaria control. The API declined to about

5, as reflected by figure 5.11, but this can be reduced further.

TB Control: The main objective of this programme was to achieve complete detection and treatment of cases. The postcard system was used to follow-up tuberculosis patients. The number of patients who completed the treatment increased from 48 to 62 per cent, and the lost rate declined from 31 to 5 per cent during a fifteen-year period. SR also successfully introduced Directly Observed Treatment under Supervision (DOTS) strategy in 1996.

FAMILY PLANNING

This programme forms the main part of the government PHC. Though SR recognizes that population control is an important issue, it feels that the quality of other health care programmes and awareness is important in order to provide better family planning (FP) services. SR has integrated this programme into other important programmes like maternal and child health, immunization, and curative services.

The programme has created a fair level of awareness among the people on various methods of FP and has gained acceptance over the years. A special programme for newlyweds was also introduced to sensitize them about aspects of reproduction and the importance of spacing. The couples themselves started coming forward to accept one of the family planning methods. SR also observed that the couples prefer to undergo sterilization operations once they have their desired number of children. The preference for a son still continues.

In 1995-6, SR devised a method of setting its own targets for internal monitoring based on ground realities and the felt needs of the eligible couples. It took into consideration the current birth rate, the Couple Protection Rate (CPR), child patterns, and couples' preferences when setting targets for various FP methods. These targets were generated by the workers themselves, which helped them to own the responsibility of achieving them. The targets were assigned to an entire sub-centre team rather than to an individual worker.

As a result, SR has been able to maintain a CPR of about 69 per cent and a birth rate of about 21 since 1995-6—the goal which was to be achieved under HFA by 2000. The mean number of children for couples accepting a permanent contraceptive method was around 2.7, which is significantly less than other government PHC areas. Even among spacing methods, the emphasis was put on continuation of the method by couples rather than on the number of new couples using the methods. This put the emphasis on behaviour change rather than on target numbers.

In addition, SR started an infertility clinic in 1997 and a senior Obstetrician and Gynaecology specialist comes from Vadodara to this clinic on a weekly basis. In general, more than 100 new couples are availing themselves of these services, and 10 couples are benefiting every year.

MAKING A DIFFERENCE: INFLUENCING FACTORS AND PROCESSES

The government has its own fixed systems, and SR had to work within this system and its requirements. With the support, time, and energy of key government functionaries who supported collaboration, it took the government nearly five years to appreciate the transparency, flexibility and innovations of SR. Once the government accepted the principle of flexibility, the modalities were required to be built in so SR has been working within the government system for the last ten years but has been able to achieve comparatively better utilization of its services and better health status in the project areas. It has been able to achieve this because of several managerial, technical, and process innovations introduced into the programme.

DECENTRALIZED TARGET SETTING, PLANNING AND MONITORING

The health workers, in consultation with beneficiaries and the community, set the targets at SR. Unlike the government's system of setting a standard target for all PHCs, SR decided yearly targets by using certain criteria and by looking at ground realities.

For example, an area's previous year's birth rate is an important basis for setting the MCH programme target. Similarly, family planning targets are set based on identifying eligible couples and their specific needs rather than generalizing targets for an entire group of couples together.

GOVERNMENT GRANTING RELAXATIONS AND FLEXIBILITY FOR . . .

- Recruitment criteria.
- Introduction of user's fees.
- Delivery Pack.
- Medicines during health camps.
- Allowing flexibility in programme prioritization.
- Routine health check-up of ICDS and school-going children by workers themselves instead of doctors.
- Strategy of orientation training camps changed.
- Sub-centre as a unit and joint responsibility by male and female workers.
- Integration of ICDS and PHC supervisors.
- Target setting and planning by workers.
- Separate reporting and monitoring system granted for SR PHC.
- No direct control and supervision of SR PHC staff by government.

Similarly, SR has decentralized monitoring. The teams themselves analyse and review the work line. At SR, when targets are not achieved, the search for where what went wrong, and why rather than who is responsible is conducted. The figures are used for understanding successes and failures. The workers link each numeric figure to the people in the field. The exercise helps the workers make changes in their field approach and ensures greater effectiveness. This helps to significantly increase the workers' involvement and helps form a positive reputation for the programme within the community. Such monitoring systems are not seen in the government where the figures are simply to be achieved and reported to the higher authorities. Achieving targets is linked to employee promotions, and it puts pressure on the workers to report incorrect information.

INNOVATIVE INTERVENTIONS

- Distribution of pre-sterilized delivery packs to mothers.
- *Dai* incentives for high-risk referral target setting in family planning.
- Team effort in target achievement.
- Once-a-week operative camps on a scheduled day.
- Involvement of field workers in target setting exercises based upon ground realities and micro-planning.
- Comprehensive MIS.
- Reporting in a single format rather than multiple and overlapping formats.
- Reporting from a sub-centre as a unit rather than as an individual worker reporting.
- Recording service utilization under the heads of project and non-project beneficiaries.
- Experimentation with impregnated mosquito bed nets for malaria control.
- Use of SR's video *Kali Kem Mari* in several government training programmes for health workers at first referral units under safe motherhood initiative.
- Recognition of SR centre for posting/training of—
  - Intern doctors
  - Female health workers
  - PHC medical officers.

MOTIVATION-CUM-MONITORING MEETINGS

Apart from annual target setting and monitoring, SR has developed a schedule for meetings at various levels. The main purpose of these meetings is to provide on-going training, motivation, problem identification, problem solving, and experience sharing, which creates an environment conducive to learning. While sharing experiences and incidents from the field, the workers not only share the good points but also admit their lapses. Again, this is encouraged not as a *fault finding* but as a *fact finding* process used for problem solving and learning from each other. The staff is also provided continuing education and training on relevant issues and diseases. Emphasis is always on handling critical cases and learning from those who have died.

A TYPICAL MEETING OF CHP STAFF AT SR INCLUDES . . .

- A prayer and inspirational reading.
- Appreciation of an individual's good performance: Learning from both positive field experiences and any shortcomings as shared by workers themselves.
- Difficulties and problem solving.
- Session on the continuing education.
- Performance review and planning for the next month by respective sub-centre teams.
- Review of critical cases and deaths in the field.
- Replenishment of medicines and other supplies.

Report System

SR has prepared its own user-friendly records and formats for programme reporting. Sub-centre teams at the village level maintain a register each day. This information is aggregated in a single reporting format every month by the village and by the sub-centre, which is then aggregated at the PHC/ICDS level at SR. This has reduced paper work and duplication of reports and information. Moreover, the workers find it easy to monitor and review their own activities and to find out where they have succeeded and failed.

Integration of PHC and ICDS and Uniform Cadre of Supervisors

To bring about managerial efficiency, SR has integrated the activities of these two programmes. SR recognizes that the two programmes need to complement each other rather then work separately. It has redefined the tasks and responsibilities of the female and male workers, TBAs, AWWs, and supervisors to avoid conflicts. This helps them to work as a team to achieve common goals.

At SR, both male and female health workers are given distinct geographical areas, populations (4-5 villages), and clearly defined responsibilities. The AWWs and *dais* are an integral part of this team. Since 1992-3, the tasks of male and female health supervisors and of *anganwadi* supervisors have been integrated with one person taking responsibility for only two sub-centre teams (consisting of *dais*, *anganwadi* workers, and health workers). Appropriate training is provided to them with the help of technical consultants. All of these measures have helped in reducing supervisor field areas and avoiding duplication, confusion, and conflict at the grassroots level.

Convenient Timing for Service Delivery

Preparing service time schedules convenient for communities has contributed to effective utilization of provided services. SR provides services at times most convenient to the beneficiaries and not to the organization itself. This is particularly important for house visits for curative, maternal, vaccination, and *anganwadi* services.

Information Dissemination

The organization effectively uses blackboards at the sub-centres and public notice boards for displaying event information, HW visits, and special medical visits to the village. The sub-centre notice boards also display the targets, which are updated monthly, to be achieved under each programme. The sub-centre charts display the number of children in different age groups, the names of pregnant women and their dates of delivery, and vaccination information.

Strengthening of Village Functionaries

All the villages have at least one trained *dai* and an AWW who are available round the clock. Efforts have been made to strengthen these local-level functionaries by providing task-specific training, including treatment of minor ailments. Ongoing support, guidance, and performance-based incentives are the key towards building such a cadre of workers. SR has experienced that strengthening this cadre of grassroots workers is the answer to providing quality primary health care at the village level. In this way, the community has also become more self-reliant. This has not only enhanced worker capacity, credibility, and self-esteem, but has also made middle-level workers free to concentrate on more technical and speciality tasks.

Referral Services

SR has developed a referral system which links village-level health care to the hospital. Referral slips are given to all the village workers. In case the village workers are not able to provide treatment for the ailment, they fill out a referral slip and gave it to the patient with all the details, including the patient's economic condition. The slip when presented at the hospital helps the doctor in providing better treatment to the patient. After the patient is discharged from the hospital, the slip is returned to the field-level workers with information about the diagnosis, treatment given, and follow-up advice. The paramedical workers and village-level workers then follow-up the case in the field. This has greatly helped in building the credibility of the field workers among the community and also enhanced health workers' confidence in providing village-level treatment. It has also turned out to be a very effective tool for auditing field and hospital services.

Postcard System

The postcard system is a process where postcards are mailed to patients to remind them of follow-up visits that they need. It was first used by the organization to follow-up tuberculosis patients, and is now being used for high-risk mothers, newborns, and tubectomy follow-ups. This system has helped workers carry out the government programme with more confidence and has helped them view patients as persons to be provided care and not as targets to be reached.

Pictorial Growth/Monitoring Cards

SR has developed pictorial cards regarding ANC and PNC awareness for illiterate mothers. Such cards are also developed for growth monitoring of young children and for key information regarding child health. Another health awareness card regarding sickle cell disease and consequent marriage prospects with colour codes was developed for persons having sickling positivity.

USING $CUSO_4$ FOR TESTING HAEMOGLOBIN (HB) LEVEL

SR introduced copper sulphate ($CUSO_4$) solution for testing Hb levels at the field level. By using this method, the result is made available immediately. The workers carry $CUSO_4$ solution of different concentrations. A drop of blood is placed in the solution, and the person can see for himself whether the drop of blood floats or sinks in the solution. If the blood sinks, then it is considered to be heavy and within normal limits. If the blood stays at the top, it is considered to be light, and the person understands that he was anaemic. This has helped workers start and monitor iron and folic acid supplementation effects and, if need be, to refer the patient to the hospital.

DELIVERY PACK

One of SR's major inputs is the development of a delivery pack for facilitating safe home deliveries. In use since 1987, it is a disposable pack to be used only once. It contains essential instruments and equipment required by birth attendants. It is compact, pre-sterilized, and has a long shelf life. These delivery packs are given during the third trimester to pregnant women when they are preparing for childbirth. The pack carries pictorial information about the contents and how they are to be used. So apart from trained *dais*, these packs are designed to be used even by the illiterate and they have contributed greatly in helping to conduct home delivery aseptically.

It is encouraging to note that the government of Gujarat has decided to introduce such delivery packs throughout the state.

OTHER INNOVATIONS

Some of the innovations tried out include providing malarial prophylaxis during pregnancy, giving vitamin A supplements to mothers after delivery, and the use of mosquito nets.

COMMUNITY PARTICIPATION

Community participation can be looked at through the community's relationship with the organization, community access to services, and the community's control over these services. With more than 15 years of experience in community health, SR realized that if good quality services are made available on an ongoing basis, people would come forward to contribute in ways described below:

1. Contribution of resources to AWWs and maintenance of health posts. Donation of land and provision of labour for the construction of health posts.
2. Support in organizing health education programmes or trainings in the village.
3. Utilization of services provided by the organization, which reflects the acceptance and support of the organization.
4. Use of emergency hospital services during serious ailments and preventive care. Delivery cases are referred to the SR hospital. Feedback is provided on the quality of the services.
5. Community support when SR wanted to use new technologies and new products such as the delivery pack and the vector control malaria programme at the field level with the village panchayat and the community.
6. Participation of the community in meetings that are held for target setting, planning, monitoring, and evaluation.

However, it was realized that long sustained community involvement in preventive health is too much to expect with many immediate pressing health problems, particularly among disadvantaged sections.

Introduction of programme content and structure was possible because of a series of micro-level interventions (Annexure 9.4) and innovations such as convenient timings and designated days for service delivery, ensuring curative care (felt need of the community), strengthening village-based health volunteers, integration of ICDS and PHC staff, use of pre-sterilized delivery packs for home deliveries, making sub-centres into team units, involvement of all levels of workers in target setting and micro-planning, and simplified MIS. It also highlighted that with appropriate reallocation of funds, it is possible to effectively manage PHCs with the present resources.

LIMITATIONS AND CONSTRAINTS

There were many expected and unexpected limitations faced by SR, some of which could be solved while some remained unresolved. They are briefly described below.

- SR felt that community participation remained limited in the project for several reasons. With total health care responsibility, the scope for bargaining with the community was limited as all the health services were supposed to be delivered free of cost. SR realized that health is not a priority to people unless there is an emergency or acute illness. Community involvement could not be sustained for preventive health measures. The pressure of target achievements also hampered the process. SR felt that collaboration with the government accentuated the magnitude of this problem.
- There are areas of public health which may not be considered part of primary health care, but directly or indirectly affect people's health. These public health areas include drinking water provision, sanitary latrine construction, smoking/tobacco/masala chewing addictions, alcohol addictions, and cancer control measures.
- Nothing concrete could be done to involve local practitioners such as *bhagat bhuvas* or to integrate allopathy with traditional medicines.
- SR experienced a few major constraints in working with the government specifically as listed below:
    - There was an overemphasis on quantitative targets at the expense of quality performances.
    - There were frequent delays in the release of grants.
    - SR felt that sincere and serious efforts to involve other voluntary organizations in replicating this PHC management experiment were lacking.

- Whenever there was a transfer of senior district officers, it required repetitive meetings to orient them about aspects of such collaborative experiments.
- It was observed that, unknowingly, over a period of time some of the SR functionaries themselves became bureaucratized following a change of their own mindset due to working with the government.

LESSONS LEARNED AND THE SCOPE FOR UPSCALING/REPLICATION

These ten years of experience have provided insight into a number of issues. The learning is primarily found in areas of NGO-GO collaboration. Secondly, there are more insights about innovations introduced in various health systems and programmes, building referral linkages, and, most importantly, the process of motivating staff in spite of working within the government infrastructure.

SUGGESTIONS FOR FOSTERING NGO–GO PARTNERSHIP

- *Willingness to Understand and Appreciate*: Both the government and the NGO must be willing to understand and appreciate the basic value systems and strengths of the other and be ready to work in the true spirit of partnership.
- *Principle of Accountability*: Both parties must observe this aspect. For example, the voluntary organizations need to send financial and functional reports regularly, and the government should be accountable to the voluntary sector in terms of timely sanctions and release of grants and other items on an ongoing basis.
- *Flexibility and Relaxation*: After ascertaining credibility, efficiency, and transparency, there is a need to give flexibility in areas such as recruitment criteria, implementation strategies, allowing user fee from affordable patients, reallocation of budgetary heads, programme prioritization, and reporting and monitoring systems.
- *Preserving the Innovative Nature of the Voluntary Organization*: Voluntary organizations have an inherent nature of

innovation and experimentation and can develop alternative models and methods that are suitable to the people, giving specific attention to the socio-cultural, educational and economic condition of the community. The government needs to recognize this role of voluntary organizations and encourage them by giving them the freedom to take up innovative PHC programmes on an experimental basis. It requires the relationship to be non-patronizing and in the true spirit of collaboration and partnership.

- *Government Sensitivity*: The government needs to be sensitive about the self-respect and dignity of voluntary organizations and needs to give organizations more autonomy. A different mindset is necessary for more involvement by communities and voluntary organizations.
- *Reallocation of Funds*: Financial viability is a major issue in the replication of any service programme. It was observed that SR's overall PHC expense equal that of the government budget if SR was allowed to replace the same amount of money saved from salaries and allied heads, to pay for the purchase of medicines, transportation, stationary, maintenance of equipment, and strengthening village-level workers. Hence, the SR experiment demonstrated that if reallocation of budgetary heads was allowed at the local level with organized and decentralized planning and management, efficient service delivery by a PHC could be ensured within the existing financial allocations.
- *Influencing at Policy/Planners Level*: In order to make NGO-GO collaboration effective, influencing at the policy/planner level is crucial. Moreover, the spirit of partnership also needs to pervade to all the levels.

Lessons Learned within the System

- *Strengthening the Village Level Worker*: In one of the operational research studies conducted by SR, it was proved that with proper training, support, guidance, ongoing monitoring and performance-based incentives, the team of village-level health volunteers could successfully deliver almost all the general functions of a full-time female health worker.

- *Referral Linkages*: The outreach primary healthcare programme and referral hospital services are both essential and complementary to each other. This referral system plays an important role in fulfilling the community's felt need for curative care and in handling complicated cases.

- *Building Team Spirit Among Staff Members*: As more and more powers and responsibilities like target setting, activity monitoring, etc., are delegated to workers, they develop a sense of involvement in decision-making and ownership of the programmes and its results.

- *Influencing the Younger Generation*: Efforts need to be made to provide an encouraging environment, guidance, support and role models whom they can look up to.

- *Other Effective Innovations*: These include extensive use of delivery packs for home deliveries, training and involvement of village-level workers, motivation and mobilization of the entire staff, referral linkages, health education sessions in villages, and so on.

CONCLUSION

It is encouraging to note that the Government of Gujarat has shown a willingness to introduce some of the effective SR interventions into their larger government system. Examples of these are pre-sterilized delivery packs, fixed days for different services, simplified MIS with the sub-centre as a unit, involvement of workers in micro-planning and target-setting exercises, strengthening the cadres of grassroot workers, and so on.

Moreover, it is inspiring to note that the Karnataka government has also successfully experimented with a few NGO-GO partnership models in recent years. Moreover, the Government of Gujarat has also entrusted voluntary organizations with the responsibility of managing three CHCs and one PHC. All these initiatives are following the International Conference on Population and Development (ICPD) in Cairo in 1994, the introduction of a Reproductive and Child Health (RCH) initiative at national and state levels, and the experiences of the SR model.

Since there has been a stagnation in Indian social indicators for several years, and the government health services are falling behind, there is an obvious need to bring about critical changes in the approach and strategy for improving the quality and coverage of primary health care services, particularly for interior and rural areas. Community initiatives, involvement of voluntary organizations, strengthening of village level workers, decentralization of health care delivery, among other measures, will make a substantial difference. This review, detailing the process as well as achievements of a PHC-managed by SEWA Rural, will provide considerable impetus and momentum in that direction.

ANNEXURE 9.1

EVOLUTION OF COMMUNITY HEALTH PROJECT 1982-2004

Particulars	*1982-4*	*1984-9*	*1989-99*	*From 1999 Onwards*
Extent of Govt. Collaboration	Village-level health worker's responsibility (CHVs, AWWs, *Dais*)	Total health responsibility – Functional PHC	Formal PHC recognition	• First Referral Unit· • Family centred safe motherhood and newborn survival
Coverage	10 villages (11,000 population)	39 villages (35,000 population) (84-21 villages, 89-39 villages)	31 villages (40,000 population)(including Jhagadia headquarter)	180 Villages 1.83 lakh Population Whole Jhagadia Block
Health Services/ Programmes	• Mobile dispensary • Maternal care • Immunization • Health education • TB follow-up	(A) Preventive, curative and promotive health care including MCH, family planning, control of malaria, TB, school health, etc. (B) Ref. services	(A) Total health care Responsibility (B) Referral hospital (C) Field operational research studies (D)Training	(A) Improving the referral support for complicated maternal and newborn cases of whole taluka. (B) To strengthen Em. OC (C) Training
Infrastructure	Three-Tier System (A) Village level Workers 1:700/1000	Four-Tier System (A) Village Level Workers: 700/1000	Four-Tier System (A) Village level Workers: 700/1000	(A) 300 *Dais* 1:700/ 1,000-1,204 orientation and monitoring

(Contd.)

ANNEXURE 9.1 (Contd.)

Particulars	*1982-4*	*1984-9*	*1989-99*	*From 1999 Onwards*
	1. *Anganwadi* workers & helpers 2. Traditional birth attendants (*Dais*) 3. Community health volunteers (CHV) (B) Mobile dispensary 1. Doctor 2. Nurse 3. Compounder (C) Referral hospital	(B) Middle level 1. Mobile dispensary 2. Male & female health workers 1:3,000/5,000 3. Health supervisors1:12,000/ 15,000 (C) Primary Health Centre 1:40,000 (D) Referral hospital 1:2,00,000	(B) Middle level 1. Male & female health workers 1:3,000/5,000 2.Health supervisors 1:12,000/15,000 (C) Primary Health Centre 1:40000 (D) Referral hospital 1:2,00,000 (E) Research & training centre	*Anganwadis* (B) 5 *Anganwadi* Supervisors, 1:20,000 health supervisors 47 Sub-centre/FHWS 35 MPHWS(C) 7 PHCs 1:40,000(D) 2 CHCs 1:2,00,000(E) 1 FRU 1:2,00,000
Funding	Oxfam (UK) Community Aid Abroad (Australia)	Govt. of India/USAID Govt. of Gujarat/Dist. Panchayat, Bharuch	Govt. of Gujarat/ Dist. Panchayat, Bharuch Ford Foundation	Govt. of Gujarat/ Dist. Panchayat Bharuch UNICEF Macarthur Foundation

ANNEXURE 9.2

HIGHLIGHTS OF THE 1989 GOVERNMENT RESOLUTION FOR TAKING OVER A PHC

- At the first stage, the management of the PHC at Jhagadia was entrusted to SR for ten years.
- The state government agreed to finance the entire PHC services in the SR project area. The service would be run on the same lines as that of the government but managed entirely by SR.
- The organization was required to fulfil all targets set by the government for various health services.
- District Panchayat (DP) Bharuch will take over the management of the PHC if the organization either does not want to manage the PHC at the end of the project or discontinues its activity.
- The organization could accept employees from DP on deputation. If the organization wants to recruit the employees on its own selection process, it can do so by following the recruitment resolution of the concerned vacancy of either government or the DP whenever possible.
- When the organization wants to appoint the employee by following its own criteria the organization is required to have either District Health Officer (DHO) or District Development Officer (DDO) in the selection committee.
- Whenever the collaboration is discontinued, the government will try to absorb the employees appointed by the organization provided they satisfy the necessary recruitment criteria like age limit and educational qualifications at the time of their appointment in SR.
- Similarly, whenever the collaboration is discontinued, the employees appointed by the organization who do not fulfill the recruitment criteria will be absorbed by the organization in their other activities.

ANNEXURE 9.3

ACHIEVEMENTS AT A GLANCE (SEWA RURAL PHC)

Parameters	*1982-3**	*1984-5*$^{\Delta}$	*1988-9*$^{\Delta}$	*1994-5*$^{\Delta}$	*1999 2000*$^{\Delta}$	*Gujarat Rural 99*$^{+}$	*Health for All HFA by 2000*$^{+}$
Villages Covered	11	21	39	30	30	–	–
Population	11,000	18,768	35,706	38,637	40,213	–	–
CBR	30.0	22.7	27.0	22.0	19.92	27	21
CDR	12.7	8.6	12.5	8.9	8.33	8.8	9
MMR	N A	6.2	5.3	4.6	00	4-6?	<2
IMR	172	81	89	62	41	70	<60
NMR	–	63.0	45.7	43	24	45	35
CPR (per cent)	37.0	55.2	61.8	69.5	71.2	56.6	60
Antenatal Care (per cent)	< 25	44	75	76	91	–	85
Institutional Delivery per cent	–	<10	16	24	35	21.8	–
Delivery Conducted by Trained Person (per cent)	20	80	90	86	93	–	–
Postnatal Care (per cent)	<25	NA	NA	95	96	–	–
Prevalence of Vitamin A deficiency	High	High	Moderate	Low	Low	–	–

Babies with Birth Weight <2.5kg (per cent)	N A	N A	N A	66	47	–	10
Severe PEM (per cent)	16.0	15.3	11.5	1.8	2.5	–	–
DPT (per cent)	<10	44	89	92	99	–	85
Measles (per cent)	N A	25	73	91	98	–	85
Epidemics of Measles, Diarrhoea Whooping Cough, etc.	Frequent	Frequent	Sporadic	Sporadic	Sporadic	Sporadic	Sporadic

Notes: * Baseline survey

Δ In-service records

+ Basic Health Statistics Gujarat, 2000-2001

ANNEXURE 9.4

LIST OF INTERVENTIONS

- Emphasis on availability of curative care for minor ailments at village level, 1982-3
- Fixing convenient times and places for service delivery, 1984-5
- Strengthening of *dais*, 1984-5
- Use of delivery packs, 1987
- Performance-based incentives to *dais*, 1989-90
- Care of unmarried pregnancies, 1987-8
- Special care for high-risk mothers, 1989-90
- Adolescent girls' health and development, 1989-90
- HB estimation—filter paper method, 1990-1
- Vitamin A supplementation in postnatal period, 1990-1
- Postcard system for follow-up of family planning, high-risk pregnancy, TB patients, etc., 1990-1
- Postnatal care within one week, 1990-1
- Sub-centres as a team unit, for planning, monitoring, and supervision tasks, 1992
- MIS system to reduce duplication of records
- Common supervisors—integration on ICDS and PHC staff, 1992
- Decentralization process—involvement of workers in target setting, monitoring, etc., 1993-4
- Programme for newly married couples, 1993-4
- De-worming and malaria prophylaxis during pregnancy, 1993-4
- Payment for delivery packs, 1993-4
- Management of ARI by AWWs, 1993-4
- Quality care of pregnant mothers with a total of three ANC check-ups (one at < 16 weeks, one at 24-8 weeks, and one after 36 weeks, 1994-5
- Blood donation camps in villages, 1994-5
- HB estimation, $CUSO_4$ method, 1994-5
- Infertility programme, 1994-5
- RTI treatment at sub-centre level by FHWs, 1994-5
- Special packages for newborn care, 1996-7

CHAPTER 10

For Whom the Reform Tolls?

ALAIN VAGUET

Health sector reforms is a recurrent theme across the world; irrespective of the level of development of nations. The worst situations, in term of life expectancy, are worth a revolution, but it seems clear that health sector is as much an economic and a political concern as strictly a health one.

For some critics, health care reform engineers 'simply reproduce themselves rather than bring about effective change'. In that case, health sector reforms 'appears as a defensive mechanism aiming to prolong the survival of the dominant system of health care',[1] in short, a protection invented by the main actors to sustain their professional interests. Other authors, more optimistic, considered that a lot has been accomplished in the European region over the last decade by incremental reforms.[2]

The most pertinent questions therefore are: Whom does the reform cure? Is this worldwide tendency wanted by civil society (bottom-up)? Does it reflect a political will, orchestrated by powerful lobbies of globalization (top-down)? We will select some arguments taken from European health systems to show the broad tendencies and their results. Finally, we will draw some conclusions on the position of India.

HOW FAR IS HEALTH ATTRIBUTABLE TO THE HEALTH SECTOR?[3]

Some researchers doubt that health systems are very much responsible for the health status of the populations. According to them, the correlation is limited to morbidity and crude number of General Practitioners (GP), or percentage of national GDP devoted to health. This argument draws us to the debate opened by Dubos,[4] and Illich,[5] who showed that health does not rely merely on the number of medicals, or sophisticated techniques, but mostly on socio-political factors. Today, this opinion is widely shared, even by the World Health Organization. If the population of developed countries could experience a long life span, it's because they are globally and individually rich and not only because health expenditure is high. But at the same time, as economists have showed, the level of spending concerning health is highly correlated with the general level of wealth of a society. It means that health is considered as a high social value, some spoke of 'modern totem' to qualify it. This explains the compulsion of citizens toward the consumption of health products and the acceptance of high-level individual and collective expenses. But where is the limit?

Without any reform comes the commodification[6] of health. That means making hospital and health products more attractive, through marketing and advertising. The end result is that health care users are treated as consumers. That is one of the determinants which can explain why the richest countries do not experience the best life expectancy. Health budget is an important point, but obviously, the political system interferes. So, the fifteen countries of the European Union (79 years) and Japan (81.5 years), registered better results than the USA (77 years). This difference is widening although the spending per head is higher (at least twice) in the latter. In fact, the experiences of Japan or Nordic countries reveal that if the social class differences are lower, better are the life expectancies.

In this context, a lot of social scientists[7] consider the right to health as mostly rhetoric. If we remember that the principal determinants of health status are not medical,[8] why should we accept to spend more on health budget instead of improving the life conditions of the poorest?

The same paradox arises when global institutions try to finance rapidly the fight against major diseases such as AIDS or TB. The scaling up of health investments in developing countries faces bottlenecks like lack of infrastructure and of professionals. For reforms too, funding remains necessary but it can't substitute a strong political will. The following examples show that the first priority of most health system reforms is budget concern, instead of health concern.

REFORMS MADE TO SUSTAIN HEALTH SYSTEMS

We can trace a common concern in the history of post-World War II states toward the concern for protection against ageing (pension) and illness, but it is important to point out that the philosophies prevailing in the diverse options remains very different in each state. Broadly speaking, in the developed world, we can trace three models depending upon cultural and political choices.

- Liberal systems, as in the United States and South America. They are financed up to 40 per cent by the public sector for Medicare-Medicaid, 30 per cent by private insurance and the remaining 30 per cent by customers.
- National systems (State managed) funded by taxes, as in north and south Europe, Canada, Australia (and India at the time of the constitution Bhore Committee, 1950).
- Compulsory health insurance (managed market) funded by workers and their enterprises, as in Germany, France and Japan.

This typology reflects social and political values and it is hard to judge them in terms of health status results.

On the other hand, national health systems (NHS) always have a better control on health budget (7 per cent of GDP in UK or 8.7 per cent in Sweden) than liberal (14 per cent in USA) and health insurance (10 per cent in France) systems. That is why, many economists conclude that NHS is the best system. But a lot of medical professionals doubt the quality of service offered under NHS. Everyone knows the long waiting list of non-urgent operations in the UK.

On the contrary, compulsory health insurance systems promote the freedom of patients and of stakeholders, but the cost of such comfort and quality is uncontrolled budget. Thanks to the enormous spending, the liberal system remains technically excellent, but the health status of persons and access are very unequal.

In fact the best results are found in northern Europe, as in Sweden, where more than 85 per cent of the spending are covered by the system. In France the score is only 60 per cent, which explains why more than 85 per cent of the French (against 1 per cent Swedish and 11 per cent of British) have got an additional private health insurance for health cost not covered under the national funding. But numbers are not enough to give a complete idea of the service, or of its capacity to take care of patients.

If between states the difference of wealth is controlled, their results in terms of life expectancy can be broadly compared. But today each system is facing a financial crisis due mostly to costly improvements in medical sciences and only secondly due to population ageing. So, reforms are mainly organized to make these systems sustainable in economic terms. Both people and health professionals are anxious or reluctant to any change. The former are afraid to pay more 'out of pocket', the latter are afraid of reduction in earnings.

In the given context, the reforms-driven regulation of spending is of two types.[9] In the USA, 'managed care' introduced the law of markets. Industrialists fund their employees' private insurances, so they decided to reduce the consumption of medical services. For the same reason, insurance companies themselves who are largely in charge of the system try to refrain all medical spending. For this purpose, call centres were created to advise patients without any visit to a professional (do it yourself); access to specialists was restricted by the compulsory referral of a GP. New kinds of medical practices such as ambulatory services reduced the number of hospital beds (up to one-third in Canada). Medicines are now purchased in large quantities after negotiations with the pharmaceutical industry and sent by post in order to cut the cost (25 per cent in USA). In the same way, after the development of medical information system, the staff of the hospital had access to information concerning patients. So, the staff can decide if an operation is necessary. From individual, the work became collective. The practitioner is under supervision, and can even be evicted.

In the managed care, MCOs (Managed Care Organizations) such as insurance companies increasingly interfere in the medical domain in order to make the system sustainable. From the point of view of geographers, it may be noted that the market-driven system always leads to uneven development and lack of territorial justice.

The second form of regulation—that of the state—seen mainly in the UK has produced competition between health providers. Hospitals have now to attract patients, otherwise they may be closed. In the same way, with the revolution of fund holdings, the authorities gave a new responsibility to GPs: the health budget is more or less in their hands. To reduce spending, GP fund holders can, for example, negotiate the price of operation of their patients; in this way, medical practitioners themselves become purchasers (but informed purchasers).

In spite of the reforms, however, the waiting list remains. For this reason, and contrary to the general trend, the New Labour decided to increase income taxes in order to improve the system rapidly (first class service), including the promotion of some private partnership.

The State here controls the power of professionals. On the contrary in France the system is free control. Everyone is free, patients and professionals. It is thus a very expensive health system where the power of practitioners is high. In terms of location the professionals concentrate in well-off cities, especially in the South of France and in the capital, while small towns lack basic services. Professionals try to increase the number of medical students, but this number is under State regulation. The government hesitates to introduce real reforms. The French almost seem allergic to managed care but how long will this option survive?

As we saw, a health system is an ideological construction; it produces a specific balance of power between different stakeholders. Even in the context of the European Union, it is very hard to transfer any innovation in governance from a state to another. Attempts to reduce inflation budgets are always partially unsuccessful. For example, in France, any attempt to regulate the price of a medical visit or the price of medicines is rapidly thwarted. Professionals adjust their strategies rapidly to maintain their earnings (increase number of consultations and prescriptions). On the other side, when the control of the State is strict, as in the UK, the population criticizes the level and quality of health offer.

It may be clear to the reader that the *scaffolding* of national health systems has a long internal history. All these national health systems have evolved over the years. For that reason, they remain largely independent and the transfer of innovation, reforms and so one, are difficult. But in the long term they are not totally closed to each other.

THE FRENCH, GERMAN AND BRITISH MODELS

In France, the present system was born after the Second World War. But social protection can be traced back to before the French Revolution when professional corporations or churches were in charge. Slowly in the nineteenth century the role of the State began to emerge, trying to reach the ideal of the Revolution: assistance to the poorest, in all the circumstances of their life, to restore their dignity.

The 'Sécurité Sociale' was created in 1945-6 and, as its promoters said it was not a reform but a revolution. The compulsory solidarity of all workers could offer a replacement earning in case of disease and reimburse the cost of medical treatment. In fact Sécurité Sociale followed similar systems set up in Germany and United Kingdom earlier. In fact, the Beveridge report of 1942 in the UK was crucial and influenced the French system. It should also be pointed out that the French decision to finance the health sector by contribution from workers and not by revenue taxes as in the UK, was on the lines of what Chancellor Bismarck introduced in Germany in the late nineteenth century.

The present reform in France is dated of 1996. Before that, the budget of social protection was in the hands of the representatives (trade unions) of industrialists and their employees. By the way we should remember that social protection was much more important than the entire State budget. From 1996, the legislature started to discuss the health budget annually and fixed it according to the proposal of the government.

Still unable to reduce the deficits, another major reform was introduced in 1999. The creation of 'Couverture Maladie

Universelle' (universal disease protection) extended the free medical assistance to the jobless, to immigrants and homeless. In one word, the rights to health was no more dependent upon the occupation and contribution but simply on citizenship, more or less like in the UK. This change was expected for a long by NGOs. Without any doubt this reform had an important impact on the health of the poorest. If not ideal, it created conditions to access medical offer treatment, either public or private. This reveals that conducive for the poor a rich country can afford such spending, which is not the cause of its deficit.

But how far can local powers or communities help to improve the situation?

THE EPIDEMICS OF DECENTRALIZATION

Worldwide, the new wind of reform is that of decentralization. This 'is by no means a new policy theme'.[10] Since long, a typology of various situations has been made. For instance, 'deconcentration', can be a very limited handing over of administrative responsibilities. *Delegation* is the effective transfer of power to the local level. Finally there is 'devolution' of power expressed nearly as a situation of independence. *Privatization* and market-orientations can be interpreted as special cases of devolution of power to profit-oriented enterprises.

Offering new competencies in health care to the local bodies is one of the challenges of decentralization. The votaries of decentralization assume that the benefits of proximity would overcome the problem of distance and insensitivity of said inhuman, centralized power.

Most studies on effects of decentralization show that after implementation, the decisions do not look more democratic. In fact the studies found a rising risk of inequity and 'of shifting responsibility for policy decision'.[11]

It is true that the great advantage of decentralization is the freedom to organize a lot of trials. But this seems much more difficult in European health systems than in the American one. In fact, there is not one but a patchwork of systems in the USA. A lot of their trials (Managed Care, Standard cost by pathology, Medical Information Systems . . .) are coming slowly in Europe as innovations. But at the same time, American citizens are very reluctant to accept any evolution that looks like the European model. Bill Clinton failed in this attempt, and as a result, millions of US citizens have poor access to health providers. So, being decentralized may be necessary but not sufficient.

At the other extreme, one could consider the highly centralized French system. According to the local authorities (Département, Région, Commune),[12] inflation is a good reason to fear decentralization. Most of the regions belong to the opposition and are reluctant to increase local taxes to sustain an erratic national health budget. There is also a risk to see a national level administration promoting some popular decision to be implemented at the level of departments and below. The allocation for dependant old age persons (APPA) illustrated this recently. It unexpectedly increased the pressure on local finances and finally the potential number of beneficiaries was restricted. It means that the reform was adjusted to the budget, not to the needs of the patients.

To cite another example, the 95 French Departements (created at the time of the French Revolution) fund the prevention of cancer programme (among other things), following the decentralization of the 1980s. But each Departement invests very differently, according to its own interest in the matter. Is it not a pity that the second most important cause of mortality is treated so unfairly?

Likewise, local (Departement) initiatives of professionals to promote diagnosis of breast cancer were fortunately delayed by national authorities in order to adopt a better protocol (valid for the entire nation). In its existing form, there was a great risk of causing anxiety among the general population with false positive case. The prevention programme is going on, but on a state basis, and the wisdom is not necessarily local.

One should remember that too often, actions towards health may provide good electoral returns. This attitude may lead to inappropriate decisions.

In the broad literature concerning decentralization, it is hard to escape the arguments of militants. For our purpose of independent evaluation, we selected AIDS epidemic in Europe, to check if the more decentralized states were doing better than others towards this epidemic.

Since the 1980s, the rapid spread of AIDS has necessitated urgent adjustments to keep the situation under control. There was need to react effectively and rapidly to reduce the total number of cases. Thanks to efficient and egalitarian health systems, the epidemic was better controlled in Europe compared to USA.[13]

But the statistics show clearly that the level of centralization or decentralization has no correlation with the control of the epidemic. Despite being closer, local authorities haven't shown quicker reaction. Decentralized health systems of Germany or Italy have not produced a better control than highly centralized France. Moreover, France and UK, where the system is centralized, experienced very different results: France has three times more AIDS cases than UK. This clearly shows the ability of some systems to be more pragmatic than others. The ability to contact and organize the high-risk groups, such as homosexuals and drug users, is often hard to recognize at all levels. That process was very slow in France where the epidemic became a political matter and advices were diluted and aimed at the general population instead of targetting particular groups. Forty per cent of intravenous drug users were in touch with the National Health System in the UK, while the corresponding figure for France was 3 per cent. As a result, 20 per cent of intravenous drug users were infected by HIV in France and only 1.4 per cent in the UK (1992).

In Federal Germany where the system is decentralized, it was observed that some German 'Lander' (decentralized regions) had a good capacity to experiment and rapidly gave Methadone as a substitute to the drug users (without official permission). The other regions followed them as a virtue of the decentralized system. But there was a risk: Bavaria saw discrimination against specific groups.

CONCLUSION

Considering the context of the seminar 'Health Sector Reform in India', the main question would be to clarify how helpful are comparisons in between an emerging country and the richest ones. The first temptation would be to affirm simply that everywhere, the key to health improvements depends mainly on the social level of the populations. This is contrary to the viewpoints of some scientists who believe that life expectancy of Indians will rely mostly on sophisticated technologies.[14] Of course, to some extent, the health sector may help and play a role in the health status of its population. According to T. McKeown,[15] the health sector can control around 10 per cent of the mortality level. Commodification, technical improvements and to some extent ageing of populations will increase this influence in the future.

So, if health offer itself does not explain the major part of life expectancy, the positive impact of the reforms of health systems may not be visible. Worst, some researchers argue that the epidemic of reforms, which comes from international pressure, dilutes the responsibility of States and distorts national priorities. As a result, 'for the first time in independent India, the crude death rate has remained almost unchanged over the last decade'.[16] The international pressures are not restricted to the Third World; in Eastern European countries too the programmes for macro-economic adjustments occurred. In the European Union itself, external fiscal pressures were generated by the requirements for economic convergence following the Maastricht Treaty.

During the two days of seminar on Indian health reforms, the various presentations on the different goings on could not be persuasive of their efficiency in terms of morbidity or quality of life. The same goes for Europe. After every reform, citizens can observe that they have to pay more 'out of this pockets' to keep their system going on, but contrary to India, life expectancy still increases quite rapidly.

Does this mean that reforms should be banned? No. A research on the strategies of European health care systems reform concluded that the role of the State remains central. If private commercial insurers have been introduced, 'the danger of opportunistic behaviour has required substantially enlarged regulatory effort by government'. Both competitive incentives and planning mechanisms are now incorporated and 'the language of market has been progressively replaced by terms such as contestability, cooperation and accountability'.[17] But as a final conclusion, 'the central criterion appears to be not so much whether the intervention is regulatory or market oriented in nature, but rather that it is applied to the supply side of the system'. In that, the effects of reform policies were most of the time unsatisfactory and that is a great matter of concern.

Very often, it must be remembered that more than the actual reform, the political environment in which it takes place explains the difficulties encountered. So the implementation of a successful experimentation may face major drawbacks if the key actors or the citizens do not share a common will. For example, the Indian patent act gave the opportunity, to produce medicines at low costs and to spread them all over the Third World. This act, made for another purpose (promotion of Indian pharmaceutical industry), clearly saved a lot of AIDS patients, but unfortunately few Indians. The denial of AIDS all over the world has slowed down pragmatic reform in the face of an emergency, even in decentralized nations.

In the same way, health has a cost but is not only restricted to a question of budget. Political will also interferes. In this sense, the absence of health issues in the political programmes of major Indian parties is shocking. This is in contrast to Europe, where, at the time of election, there are rigorous discussions on health. It may be due to a different level of 'healthiness'[18] of the societies, but it may also be a choice of many Indians to orient their visits towards private practitioners and corporate hospitals. Worldwide, when a society becomes richer, the need for freedom and easy access increases. But experts express doubts about the quality of poorly controlled health providers.[19]

Social scientists[20] may regret the Bhore Committee when the discourses (not the facts) were in favour of a public system; stubborn Indians remain fascinated by the shining private system. One may argue about the role of globalization,[21] which is not a reform, accuse liberalization, prove its uneven spatial development[22] but the idea still remains: emerging India is building a society as unequal as before, much more oriented toward the United States model than toward the European one. In term of health sector, there is no general system of protection in the health sector. The said public system will, at best, look more like the US Medicare, mainly for the destitute, while most of the well-off will rely upon private insurance for their health costs. Is this two-tier tendency dependent on a reform?

NOTES

1. V. Stambolovic, 'Epidemic of Health Care Reforms', *European Journal of Public Health*, vol. 13, 2003, pp. 77-9.
2. J. Figueras and B.R. Saltman, 'Building Upon Comparative Experience in Health System Reform', *European Journal of Public Health*, vol. 8, no. 2, 1998.
3. S. Curtis and A. Taket, *Health and Societies: Changing Perspectives*, Arnold, 1996, p. 173.
4. R. Dubos, *Mirage of Health*, Harper Colophan, 1979.
5. I. Illich, *Limits to Medicine*, M. Boyars, 1976.
6. E. Pellegrino, 'The Commodification of Medical and Health Care: The Moral Consequences of a Paradigm Shift from a Professional to a Market Ethic', *Journal of Medicine and Philosophy*, no. 24, 2001.
7. D. Fassin and J.P. Dozon, *Critique de la Santé Publique: une approche anthropologique*, Balland, 2001.
8. Carr R. Hill, 'Efficiency and Equity Implications of the Health Care Reforms', *Social Sciences and Medicine*, 1994, 39-49, pp. 1189-1201.
9. B. Palier, La réforme des systèmes de santé. PUF, Que sais-je ? no. 3710, 2004.
10. Curtis and Taket, 1996, p. 216.
11. Idem, p. 225.
12. Commune is one of the smallest French electoral bodies (Paris is a commune, equivalent to a tiny village). Departement (total 95) is close to an Indian district. Normandy is a region (amongst 22). Each region consists of several Departments.
13. Steffen M., *Les Etats face au sida en Europe*, Presses Universitaires de Grenoble, 2001.
14. A.P.J. Abdul Kalam and Y.S. Rajan, *India 2020: A Vision for the New Millennium*, Penguin, 1998.
15. T. McKeown, *The Modern Rise of Population*, London: E. Arnold, 1976.
16. I. Qadeer, 'Health Care Systems in Transition III. India, Part III: The Indian Experience', *Journal of Public Health and Medicine*, vol. 22, no. 1, 2000, pp. 25-32.
17. Figueras and Saltman, 'Building Upon Comparative Experience in Health System Reform', *European Journal of Public Health*, vol. 8, no. 2, 1998.

18. T. Brown and C. Duncan, *Health and Place*, December 2000.
19. *Frontline*, October 2004: Out of one million medical laboratories in India, only four were under certification, none in the public sector.
20. Rama Baru, 'Health-Sector Reform: The Indian Experience', in A.C. Twaddle, *Healthcare Reform Around the World*, Westport: Greenwood Publishing Group, 2002.
21. Alain Vaguet, 'Healthcare Systems Caught in the Twists and Turns of Globalization', in F. Landy and B. Chaudhuri, eds., *Globalization and Local Development: Examining the Spatial Dimension*, New Delhi : Manohar, 2004.
22. K.V. Narayana, 'Size and Nature of Healthcare System', in C.H. Hanumantha Rao and S. Mahendra Dev, eds., in *Andhra Pradesh Development*, Centre for Economic and Social Studies, 2003.

CHAPTER 11

Ideology and Health Sector Reforms: A State-Level Analysis

RAMA V. BARU

The process of health sector reforms is well entrenched across both developed and developing countries. The elements that are included within health sector reforms are similar but the experience of reforms across countries has been varied. In India health sector reforms have included several components and have addressed various levels and sub-systems of the health service system and the national health programmes. In this paper we provide a brief overview of the ideological and historical context within which health sector reforms were initiated globally and in India. This is followed by an analysis of the role of funding agencies in articulating these ideologies through specific projects as a part of the loans to the health sector. The influence of health sector reforms are not merely confined to structural changes in the financing and provisioning of health services but have influenced technical aspects as well. The discussion then focuses on reforms at the state level that are driven by the government and those that are externally funded.

CONTEXT OF HEALTH SECTOR REFORM

HSR is feature of the 1980s and 1990s. It is a global phenomenon and is not merely a technical intervention or a value neutral process. HSR is very firmly rooted in the neo-liberal ideological framework and based on some shared assumptions that expenditure on public systems are wasteful; public systems have been inefficient and ineffective; markets need to be given greater prominence and market principles can be introduced in public systems to make them more efficient. The ideological base of health sector reforms has been widely written and commented upon by several research scholars across different countries (Qadeer et al., 2001). The ascendancy of the neo-liberal ideology is attributed to the world recession as a result of the oil shock during the mid-1970s and later the crisis and collapse of the socialist countries. In addition the welfare state was facing a crisis in terms of under-investment and problems of bureaucratized systems that were rigid and unresponsive to people's needs and expectations. It is this larger context that provided a convenient handle for an ideological position that questioned the legitimacy of the State and proposed that markets are more efficient and effective for delivering health services. It was indeed a fact that public health service systems were affected by growing demands, rising costs and organizational structures that were hierarchical with little room for responding to felt needs. Given the labour-intensive nature of the public health services the number of personnel employed by them was large and in most countries a substantial amount of the budget was spent on salaries.

These issues were well acknowledged even before the onset of the crisis and it was widely acknowledged that the health services across the globe needed reform. The debate was ideologically divided with those who viewed health as a developmental issue where the State was a key player and others who visualized a reduced role for the State and a key role for markets. The Alma Ata document on primary health care in 1978 had come up with a design where health was seen as interrelated with development and also how health services should respond to the felt needs of the people (WHO, 1979). This global policy initiative was recognition of the failure of a purely technical approach to health issues with excessive emphasis on drugs and medical care for handling infectious diseases and other health concerns. The experiences of China, Soviet Union and other socialist countries that had addressed the basic needs of their people and had placed a great deal of emphasis on providing basic services with a well worked out referral system provided a contrast to the experiences of many European and developing countries who had mainly invested in medical care with focus on secondary and tertiary rather than primary levels of care. The Alma Ata provided a design whereby inequality, poverty and development were the core concerns that demanded the State to play a central role in order to ensure that the basic needs of the population were met.

The realization of these issues was essentially political in nature and in many developing countries it had the potential to question their inegalitarian societies. This was clearly perceived as a threat by who felt that they would lose rather than gain from this initiative. Key among these were the pharmaceutical and related companies that were dependent on the large markets of ill-health in the developing countries. The Indian government that was one of the signatories of the Alma Ata document set up a committee to review health services and provide an alternative approach to achieve 'Health for All' (ICSSR/ICMR, 1981). Therefore, if one sees reforms as bringing about change in the health service system it is important to state that there were initiatives both at the global and national levels. These were driven by values like equity, universality and comprehensiveness, but there were resistances to these approaches from within countries from sections of the ruling classes, elite, professionals and the pharmaceutical industry. At the global level sections of the American political and professional class saw the Alma Ata document as promoting socialist ideology, which directly challenged the interests of the pharmaceutical industry. These various factors affected the implementation of this approach for any meaningful reform of the health sector.

The crisis within socialist countries further weakened the defense of this approach and resulted in the strengthening of greater faith in markets rather than the State. The anti-State and pro-market stance that informed the health sector reform agenda of the 1980s and 1990s is clearly articulated in its definition and content.

CONTENT AND ELEMENTS OF HEALTH SECTOR REFORM

Health sector reforms were initiated during the 1980s and 1990s with the basic tenets of improving efficiency, effectiveness and quality of care in health services. These reforms placed a strong emphasis on restructuring public health services by contracting out of ancillary services, scaling down manpower and decentralization. In addition, reforms often presume a more dominant role for the private market in finance, provision, technology and research of health care (Berman, 1995). During this period health sector reforms tended to emphasize restructuring the role of the State for selective financing, provisioning and regulating health services.

Given these set of assumptions the elements that constitute HSR are related to financing, provisioning, personnel and management. In all these elements the emphasis is on efficiency, efficacy and quality of services. Therefore initiatives are taken to reduce public spending and ensuring expanded role for markets. As a result privatization is at the core of health sector reforms. There are several forms of privatization and these include:

- Privatization of ownership, which means that the ownership of facilities and service units is shifted from the public to the private sector. This may happen by sale of shares, voucher privatization (as in the Central and Eastern European countries), transfer to management or employees, direct sale, etc.;
- privatization of responsibility, by formal transfer of responsibility for the service to a private organization, transfer to users via abolition or reduction of service, liquidation of State-owned enterprises, liberalization and reduction of planning of the sector;
- privatization of provision through contracting out, leasing, operating concessions, management contracting, purchasing of private goods and services;
- privatization of finance through higher co-payments and user charges, or by shifting to private health insurance funds, private capital for public infrastructure investment, joint ventures with private enterprises;
- privatization through the introduction of markets (for example, competitive tendering between in-house and external contractors), creation of markets by splitting purchasers and providers or introducing greater choice for patients. (PSI, 1997: 8)

Different countries have adopted combinations of approaches as a part of health sector reform and these are seen in terms of specific initiatives that include privatization through the introduction of user fees, contracting out of services and decentralization.

An analysis of the experiences of both developed and developing countries shows that it is this set of elements that have been broadly incorporated in HSR initiatives. These sets of elements have been the dominant paradigm that has guided HSR in both developed and developing countries during the last two decades. In developed countries like the UK and Canada there have been efforts to expand the space for private insurance and introducing market elements such as managed competition as was the case in the NHS reform in UK. It is often argued that this may lead to improvements in service quality and efficiency but result in increasing pressure on health care staff and management. In developing countries several of the initiatives mentioned above have been implemented either by national governments themselves or through the conditionality tied to loans that they borrow from the World Bank. It is well acknowledged that the Bank has emerged as the single largest financier of the health sector. Other multilateral and bilateral agencies largely support the ideological basis of HSR. The Bank has played a significant role in designing and prescribing policy changes in the health sector incorporating the basic tenets of HSR. The other agencies also accept the tenets but some of them are concerned about equity and the access to the poor. Over time even the Bank has incorporated these concerns in its agenda for developing countries.

EXPERIENCE OF HSR

HSR can be viewed as a complex interplay of the prevailing ideological climate and a number of actors that shape the process of reforms. This would include actors at the global, national and local levels but who are not clearly equal players in determining the process of reform. This is because power and its articulation at all levels are complex and unequal. Therefore one would see the content and process of reform as an outcome of a 'complex process that involves the interaction between global agencies, both bilateral and multilateral that promotes ideology; the national context that creates spaces for the articulation of this ideology and the health service system implements the reforms' (Baru and Nanda, 2004). Available evidence suggests that the experience of health sector reform presents a varied picture both in terms of pace and content. These variations are dependent on the history of nations; the fiscal and infrastructural state of public health services; the growth of markets in the health services; and resistance to reforms from civil society (Baru and Nanda, 2004 and Twaddle, 2002). There are a group of countries, especially from Latin America and Africa, that are not only the first generation of reformers but their pace of reforms has been extremely rapid with little resistance either from the political class or the civil society. Erstwhile socialist countries from the eastern European region and Soviet Union have privatized their health service systems over a relatively short period of time, resulting in a number of problems. The Indian experience is different in that some of the elements of reform were already in place even in the early 1980s. Therefore privatization of health services at the tertiary level and State subsidies for tertiary private sector were initiated during the 1980s, much before the Bank started loaning to the health sector in India. During the 1990s the Bank did assume a greater role and basically the elements of HSR were inbuilt into the various projects supported by the Bank, like the primary health care project, reproductive and child health project, communicable disease control and the State health systems project for strengthening secondary-level of provisioning.

CHARACTERISTICS AND EXPERIENCES OF HSR AT THE STATE LEVEL IN INDIA

In almost all Indian states elements of health system reforms have been initiated but there are differences in the content and extent of reforms. In India, states can be broadly classified into two categories with respect to HSR. The first category consists of states like Tamil Nadu, Madhya Pradesh, and Gujarat that have initiated certain elements of reform without external assistance. The second category consists of others like Andhra Pradesh, West Bengal, Orissa, Uttar Pradesh, Karnataka, Maharashtra and more recently Tamil Nadu who have sought external resources to initiate certain elements of the reform or augment the reforms with funding from multilateral and bilateral agencies.

Tamil Nadu, Gujarat, Rajasthan and Madhya Pradesh belong to those states that have initiated reforms related to drug procurement and supply, contracting out, public-private partnerships, levying user charges and issues related to personnel. There are several forms that health sector reforms have taken in different states and these include:

- Contracting out of non-clinical services in hospitals to private agencies.
- Community health financing initiatives (as a part of alternative strategies for devolving the responsibility for paying to households).
- Devolving financial and administrative responsibilities to panchayats.
- Reform initiatives at the primary level have come largely through national programmes many of which are funded by multilateral and bilateral agencies.

Tamil Nadu was one of the first states to set up a drug procurement and supply corporation called the Tamil Nadu Medical Supplies Corporation. Karnataka, Orissa, Rajasthan and several other states have now adopted the design of this innovation. The reform process in Himachal Pradesh, Haryana and some of the newly formed states has been partially supported by agencies like DFID, EC, and DANIDA.

FINANCING

This includes mechanisms to augment finances for the health sector, like introduction of user fees; setting up of Rogi Kalyan Samiti in Madhya Pradesh, Medical Relief Society in Rajasthan and Aspatal Kalyan Samiti in Himachal Pradesh. All these work on the same principle and are restricted to secondary and tertiary levels of care. The Rogi Kalyan Samiti in Madhya Pradesh set the trend for other states to follow. It was first started in a tertiary teaching hospital in Indore and then expanded to districts and even CHCs. Intially there was a great deal of euphoria based on the Indore experience where members of civil society contributed to the RKS. However the experience has been far from even across the state.[1] The Madhya Pradesh experience was a model for several other states and prominent among them are Rajasthan and Himachal Pradesh who have set up similar bodies for augmenting resources at the secondary and tertiary levels.

In Rajasthan MRS was initiated in 1995 and was seen as a means to get additional revenue that could be used by hospitals through decentralized decision making. A separate management structure consisting of a committee consisting of official and non-official members of state, regional and district level was constituted. Its functions include providing services and using the additional resources to provide facilities like toilets, medical supplies and other amenities. The Aspatal Kalyan Samiti was set up in Himachal Pradesh in 2001 with similar objectives to the RKS and MRS. The information on how these societies are functioning and how they have improved the effectiveness of hospitals is not clear.

PUBLIC-PRIVATE PARTNERSHIPS

Handing over PHCs and urban health centres to NGOs: There are examples of contracting out of PHCs to NGOs from Andhra Pradesh, Karnataka, Gujarat, and West Bengal. In Karnataka, two PHCs were contracted out to NGOs and the experience was a mixed one. Gujarat was among the earliest states that had experimented with contracting out PHCs to NGOs. In 1984 the state government had handed over several PHCs to SEWA Rural wherein the government provided the budgetary support for the staff salaries and supplies. The NGOs had to utilize their own resources to procure any additional supplies and pay the salary of the personnel. An evaluation of these various experiences shows that the NGOs in Gujarat have faced a number of difficulties but have tried to overcome them. There are only five NGOs in Gujarat who are involved in this scheme (Arya and

Mandwal, 2006). In other states the government-NGO partnership has not worked out because the latter find it difficult to run the PHCs on the budget prescribed by the government.

Decentralization: There are varied experiences of decentralization across states but in most of them it is for getting additional resources. There is mainly deconcentration of services with inadequate financial devolution to the panchayats. Decentralization then forces communities to augment resource by tapping the community. Kerala is the only state where health care institutions up to the district level have been handed over to the panchayat. In Himachal Pradesh, panchayati raj institutions have introduced Parivar Kalyan Salahkar Samiti (PARIKAS) at three levels of the panchayati raj system. These *samitis* have representatives of the panchayat institutions at different levels and their functions are related to family welfare activities. Except for Kerala where decentralization has involved personnel under the panchayats' supervision, this has not happened in other states.

Health Personnel

Several states have introduced changes in the appointment and training of personnel. Some states have been appointing doctors on a contract basis in order to overcome the shortage of personnel in rural areas; at the peripheral level they have undertaken training for multi-skilling of paramedical workers. In Rajasthan they have started appointing even staff nurses, lab technicians and ANMs on contract basis. During the 1990s the trend across several states was shortage of paramedical personnel due to non-recruitment and a freeze on training of these workers. As a result there was and continues to be a serious move to encourage community health workers on a voluntary basis or by giving honorarium. It is the poorer states, where there is both fiscal and personnel shortage, that there is a serious move to hire medical and paramedical personnel on a contract basis. Humanpower is the backbone of the health services therefore reducing investments will have negative consequences for delivery.

Contracting Out of Ancillary Services

All states have contracted out non-medical services like laundry, security and in some cases the catering services as well. While we do know that this process has been in place for some time now there is little evidence regarding its effectiveness in terms of cost and quality.

Regulation of the Private Sector

Several states like Rajasthan, Himachal Pradesh, Tamil Nadu, Andhra Pradesh and Maharashtra have introduced bills to regulate the private sector. In addition, the movement to check the mushrooming of diagnostic centres for sex determination has resulted in legal provisions for registering such institutions. In Himachal Pradesh there is a bill called The Himachal Pradesh Paramedical Council Bill 2003 whose objective is to maintain a state register of paramedical practitioners, register them and also prescribe a code of ethics for them.

Reviews of the various elements that are broadly included under the rubric of health sector reforms across states do show similarities. At present there is some rudimentary information regarding the initiatives that have been taken but little in terms of systematic documentation, analysis and lessons learned from some of these initiatives. The Bureau of Planning within the Director General of Health Services in the Ministry of Health and Family Welfare has initiated two meetings where state health secretaries shared their experiences and subsequently they have also initiated studies on specific themes. There is a need for systematic studies to be done in order to document the process and outcomes of these initiatives. From the available information it is apparent that the reform initiatives have been largely driven by fiscal crisis and do not seem to have a plan that guides this effort. They appear more like a number of initiatives that are incremental in nature that have been cobbled together at different points in time. Thus the process of reforms at the state level clearly shows the lack of a systemic perspective to reforms. Some states are reforming secondary and tertiary levels of care and primary level is being dealt with separately. Others are

TABLE 11.1: STATE-WISE REFORM INITIATIVES IN THE HEALTH SERVICE SYSTEM

Provisioning and Support Systems

Gujarat
- Creation of block health office and grouping of CHCs
- Establishment of quality control centres and blood transfusion network

Rajasthan
- Drug policy and procurement system
- Jan Mangal Scheme and BPL Medicare Card Scheme
- Contracting of ancillary services

Uttranchal
- Integration of health and ICDS programme
- Fixed day schedule for health service delivery
- Drug procurement policy
- Contracting of ancillary services

Punjab
- Development of disease surveillance system
- Performance and quality indicators for hospitals and improvement of laboratories
- Revamping of primary health services and development of referral system
- Contracting of ancillary services
- State health systems strengthening at secondary level

Madhya Pradesh
- Revision of building construction rules
- Effective operationalization of First Referral Units (FRU)
- Rogi Kalyan Samitis at secondary and tertiary levels

Andhra Pradesh
- State health systems strengthening at secondary level
- Development of disease surveillance
- Primary level strengthening
- Contracting of ancillary services

Orissa
- State health systems strengthening at secondary level
- Drug procurement policy
- Contracting of ancillary services

Himachal Pradesh
- Aspatal Kalyan Samiti established for secondary level care

Uttar Pradesh
- State Health Systems Development Project for secondary strengthening

Tamil Nadu
- Drug procurement and supplies

- Strengthening and reorganization of primary health services

Human Resources

Appointment of staff on contractual basis (most of them)

Capacity building

- Course in anaesthesia (Orissa, Rajasthan)
- Internship training for better community health orientation (Orissa)
- Contracting appointments of medical and paramedical personnel (Orissa, Gujarat, Rajasthan, Andhra Pradesh)

Reorganization of Medical and Paramedical Personnel

- Cadre of para medical ophthalmic assistant (Gujarat)
- Formation of district cadre for paramedics (Gujarat, Orissa, Andhra Pradesh)
- Promulgation of bill to register practitioners and establishments (HP)
- Redeployment of staff (Tripura)
- Integration of ISM medical officers for national programmes (MP, Uttranchal)
- Mandatory pre-PG rural service (Orissa)
- Transfer policy for MO in remote areas (Uttaranchal)
- Delegation of powers to medical officers (Gujarat)
- Multiskilling of health personnel (Rajasthan, Orissa, Uttaranchal)

Sources: 1. Compiled from state presentations on HSR organized by the Bureau of Planning and Ministry of Health, September 2003.
2. S. Nandraj, Presentation on public-private partnership at the Workshop on India's Health System: Role of Health Sector Reforms, September 2003.
3. M. Gupta, 'State Health Systems: Orissa', ICRIER Working Paper No. 89, November 2002.

focusing only on procurement and dispensation of drugs and many of them on decentralization. In the case of states supported by international agencies it is a project approach hence there is little coordination across projects. While there is some data available on the process of reform there is little or no data to assess the impact of these reforms on the health service system or the communities.

INTERNATIONAL AGENCIES AND PROJECT-DRIVEN REFORMS

As discussed earlier there are some elements of health sector reform that are directed by the state and others that are either partially or entirely funded by multilateral or bilateral agencies.

During the 1990s the World Bank emerged as the single largest agency for foreign assistance to the health sector in India. It essentially gives 'soft loans' to the health sector with its own conditionalities. The other agencies are the EC, DFID and others like DANIDA, Swedish International Development Agency (SIDA) and GZT (German acronym for German Technical Co-operation). Typically the World Bank and most other agencies have a project approach to funding and are dealing with different levels and aspects of the health service system. The major projects funded by the World Bank include the state health systems development project for secondary-level strengthening, primary health care project, reproductive and child health project and disease surveillance and monitoring project. This section examines the process and experience of state health systems development project but recognizes that other projects like the reproductive and child health project and primary-level strengthening project have incorporated several elements of the health sector reform agenda.

The secondary-level strengthening started in 1995 with Andhra Pradesh, West Bengal, Punjab and Karnataka. Subsequently Maharashtra, Orissa, Uttar Pradesh and most recently Tamil Nadu have also got loans for the state health systems development project from the World Bank. These projects provide loans for civil works, medicines, equipment purchase, training and research.[2]

A recent evaluation of the World Bank of the first set of states provides some insights into the areas in which reform was initiated and while it states that it is 'satisfactory' it raises some significant issues for sustainability of these reforms. The objectives of the state health systems project were to: (i) improve efficiency in the allocation and use of health resources through policy and institutional development; and (ii) improve performance of the health care system through improvements in the quality, effectiveness and coverage of health services at the first referral level and selective coverage at the primary level to better serve the neediest sections of society. The project focused on the first referral level because several reviews of the trends in expenditure across levels of care observed that a disproportionately high proportion of the expenditure was on the tertiary level care. This was at the expense of first referral facilities and the fact that health facilities at the primary and first referral hospitals in the states continued to face operational deficiencies due to inefficiencies. A weak primary and first referral hospital system results in an overload on the tertiary sector—a trend seen across states.

If one reviews the outcome indicators for assessing the improvement after implementation of the health systems project they include:

- Increase in out-patient and in-patient care
- Shortening of average length of stay
- Increase in bed occupancy
- High Bed turnover rates

These were to be achieved with better infrastructure and modern technology.

A preliminary review done by the World Bank of the four states, viz., Karnataka, Punjab, West Bengal and Andhra Pradesh that have completed the project raises a number of issues that need to be studied. The investment in the secondary level of care is seen as contributing to national policy objectives such as reduction in IMR and MMR, population stabilization and controlling disease burden. This kind of a formulation assumes that more investments in hospitals alone can impact these indicators significantly. The experience of mortality declines and population stabilizations clearly indicate that the process is indeed a complex process and health institutions are just one of the inputs to affect it.[3] There is a need to recognize that this project basically is focusing on hospitals and therefore how the impact on health status is going to be established is unclear.

Even for other inputs like user fees, public-private partnerships, the role and quality of private services, impact of these projects for strengthening referral systems from primary to secondary, commitment to increase investments in health and ownership of these reforms at different levels of services, etc., need to be studied and evaluated. The evidence is either scanty or lacking as a result of which there are only a few descriptions of these projects that do not lend themselves to detailed analysis. However each of these inputs raises a number of questions that need further exploration as discussed below.

Introduction of user fees and the exclusion of the poor from paying for services have been important areas for policy debates. The real question is to what extent have these projects been 'pro-poor'? Has access to health institutions improved for them and what is their perception of it? A number of these states had initiated public-private partnerships in the health sector. There is inadequate evidence regarding the nature and experience of these partnerships in terms of its strengths and weaknesses. Linked to this is the performance of the private sector itself and to what extent these projects have addressed the regulation and quality monitoring in the private sector.

Administratively a separate governing board was created that included high-level representatives from different ministries that were associated with the project. This board was empowered to make major policy decisions and develop a broad policy outline for the project; approve the annual budget; authorize major project revisions as necessary; ratify decisions made by the steering committee (in Karnataka); formulate rules and regulations; and undertake an annual review of project implementation and monitor overall project progress. (World Bank, 2005) Here again there are questions regarding what the interaction of the board is with the existing administrative structure? What is the extent of interaction between the two? Do they effectively work parallel to each another?

For the states that have completed the projects the issue of financial sustainability is critical. This essentially means that state governments have to increase their allocations for health. The recent evaluation by the Bank has raised this as the most important issue for future sustainability. While most state governments showed strong commitment and political support for health sector reform, experience showed that the area of public financing for health was a little weak. This seems to be a serious issue for the future of these projects.

DISCUSSION AND CONCLUSION

Health sector reforms are not technical initiatives but are informed by diverse ideological positions. There have been debates at the global level regarding the need for reforms even before the current wave of health sector reforms. The Alma Ata declaration on primary health care was embedded and informed by the importance of development and concern for persisting poverty and inequalities within and across societies. The primary health care approach thus recognized the relationship between ideology, politics and health; therefore it was challenged by those who saw it as destabilizing the *status quo*.

The debate for the need to reform the health sector continued and although the primary health care approach was considerably weakened with the selective primary health care approach, nevertheless several developing countries continued to use the former as a design that could ensure a more universal, comprehensive and universal health services. During the late 1970s there was an assertion of the neo-liberal ideology that sought to limit the role of the State and create greater spaces for markets, which was informed by the assumption that the latter is more efficient than the former. These ideas took root and informed the course of health sector reforms in both the developed and developing countries. The negative experience of the early reforming countries put the pro-market lobby slightly on the defensive and a 'selective role' for the State was entertained in policy debates.[4]

The experience of health sector reforms across and within countries shows variations. In some countries many of the elements of HSR have been introduced as a result of a fiscal crisis and are incremental. The process of reform has been supported by the World Bank's lending to the health sector across several developing countries. Therefore one needs to make a distinction between countries that have been influenced by the ideology of health sector reforms in general and others who have introduced it with Bank support. In the Indian context, elements like privatization and even some user fees in the public sector were in place even in the 1970s and 1980s. Other elements like contracting out and decentralization were introduced as means of cost recovery across several states. Those states that have been implementing Bank's health projects, viz., reproductive and child health project, primary-level strengthening project, secondary-level strengthening project, etc., have elements of health sector reform built into them. The available evidence on the experience of user fees across Indian states shows variation. States like Madhya Pradesh,

Himachal Pradesh and Rajasthan showed an increase in revenue with the introduction of user fees.[5] Punjab showed an overall increase but there were tremendous variations across district hospitals—some had very low recovery rates. It is clear from all states that the revenue from user fees is only an additional income and not a substitute for public financing. There is concern about what introduction of user fees is doing to access for the poor and the very poor; however the evidence is insufficient to come to any meaningful conclusions.

A number of initiatives have been tried for public-private partnerships but the evidence is presenting a mixed picture. There is little that can be generalized since it is specific to the institutions that are in partnership, the programme for which the partnership has been entered into and the kind of terms and conditions for these partnerships. This means that how replicable and upscalable these initiatives are at different levels is an open question. Although some states have included regulating the private sector as an important element of HSR, the pace, direction and content have been wanting. The focus has largely been on regulating provisioning and not adequate attention has been paid to private interests in medical, paramedical education as well as technology and drugs. There are too many well-entrenched and conflicting interests that have to be addressed by state governments in order to be effective. Any amount of reform of public sector without addressing the private sector will be ineffective in the long run. A number of these states had initiated public-private partnerships in the health sector. There is inadequate evidence regarding the nature and experience of these partnerships in terms of its strengths and weaknesses. Linked to this is the performance of the private sector itself and to what extent these projects have addressed the regulation and quality monitoring in the private sector.

For states like Karnataka, West Bengal, Andhra Pradesh and Punjab which received loans from the Bank for strengthening their secondary level care, the financial sustainability of these reform initiatives is of real concern especially when these governments continue to be in a fiscal crisis. (GOI, 2004)

This paper has attempted to provide an overview and put together some evidence on the process of reforms. This exercise has shown the enormous gap in evidence and the need for systematic research at the level of the states to enable richer analysis. There are ideological and methodological issues that inform the process and outcome of HSR, therefore researchers in this area need to acknowledge them rather than view the HSR initiative as a value neutral process.

NOTES

1. See G. Kumar, 'Promoting Public-private Partnership in Health Services', *Economic and Political Weekly*, 19 July 2008, pp. 3041-5.
2. For a detailed discussion on the outlays within these projects see R.V. Baru, 'Health Sector Reforms and Structural Adjustment: A State Level Analysis', in Qadeer et al., eds., *Public Health and Poverty of Reforms: The South Asian Predicament*, New Delhi: Sage, 2001.
3. For a detailed discussion refer to McKeown's thesis on mortality declines. Several other scholars have furthered this thesis. For example Sheila Zurbrigg's research on decline in malarial mortality in the Punjab during the nineteenth century shows the relationship between hunger and disease.
4. Based on the evidence of the negative impact of health sector reforms in the early adjusting countries in Africa and South America, a number of public health scholars and economists raised concerns regarding the consequences of blanket privatization of health services and argued that health was not like other commodities since it is a public good with externalities. For details see Robert Evans, Antia, Banerji, Qadeer, Sen, Krishnan.
5. These are states where the private sector growth at the secondary and tertiary levels is poor. Therefore even the middle and upper middle classes who would potentially constitute the bulk of those accessing private sector are dependant on the public sector. On the other hand, Punjab has a vibrant private sector and the low recovery rates can be explained by the fact there is competition between the public and private sector for patients.

REFERENCES

Arya, G. and A. Mandwal, *A Study of Contracting-out of Health Care in India*, Hyderabad: The Futures Group Policy Project, 2006.

Baru, R.V. and P. Nanda, 'Understanding the Health Sector Reform Process in India: A Historical and Analytical Overview', paper presented at a seminar organized by CHANGE, Washington D.C., 2004.

Baru, R.V., I. Qadeer and Ritu Priya, 'State and Private Sector in India: Some Policy Options', paper submitted to Ministry of Health and Family Welfare, sponsored by WHO-SEARO, New Delhi, 2000.

Banerji, D., 'Landmarks in the Development of Health Services in India', in I. Qadeer, K. Sen and K.R. Nayar, eds., *Structural Adjustment and the Paucity of Reforms in South Asia*, New Delhi: Sage, 2001.

Berman, P., ed., *Health Sector Reform in Developing Countries: Making Health Sustainable*, Cambridge: Harvard University Press, 1995.

Gupta, M., 'State Health Systems: Orissa', ICRIER Working Paper No. 89, November 2002.

Indian Council of Social Science Research and Indian Council of Medical Research, *Health For All: An Alternative Strategy-Report of a Study Group Set Up Jointly by the ICSSR and ICMR*, Pune: Indian Institute of Education, 1981.

Iyer, A. and G. Sen, 'Health Sector Changes and Health Equity in the 1990s', in S. Raghuram, ed., *Health and Equity-Effecting Change*, Bangalore: HIVOS, 2000.

Nanda, P., 'Health Sector Reform in Zambia: Implications for Reproductive Health and Rights', Working Paper, Centre for Health and Gender Equity, Washington, 2000.

Kumar, G., 'Promoting Public-Private Partnership in Health Services', *Economic and Political Weekly*, 19 July 2003, pp. 3041-5.

Nandraj, S., 'Presentation on Public Private Partnership', at the Workshop on India's Health System: Role of Health Sector Reforms, September 2003.

Public Services International (PSI), *Public Services and Private Interests*, France: Ferney-Voltaire, 1997.

Proceedings of the State Presentations on Health Sector Reform Organized by the Bureau of Planning and Ministry of Health, September 2003.

Ramachandran, P., 'India's Health System: Role of Health Reforms', Workshop on 'India's Health System: Role of Health Sector Reforms', 4-5 September 2003.

Qadeer, I., 2000. 'Health Care Systems in Transition III, India, Part I: The Indian Experience', *Journal of Public Health and Medicine*, vol. 2, no. 1, 2000, pp. 25-32.

Qadeer, I., K. Sen, and K.R. Nayar, ed., *Structural Adjustment and the Paucity of Reforms in South Asia*, New Delhi: Sage, 2001.

Twaddle, A.C., ed., *Health Care Reform Around the World*, Westport: Greenwood Publishing Group, 2002.

World Bank, *World Development Report 1993: Investing in Health*, New York: Oxford University Press, 1993.

——, Workshop on Indian Health Systems Projects: What We have Learnt and How Can We Do Better? (Lessons and Recommendations), 15-16 June, New Delhi, 2005.

Index